GW01314706

Health**Wealth**

Feel Like A Billion Dollars Every Day Of The Week

DANIEL GRANT

What People Are Saying:

"Daniel Grant - The intelligent trainer"
Susie Orbach
Author of BODIES

"A very enlightening and useful book that will guide you and inspire you in the process of attaining optimum results from your training"
Bruno Tonioli
Strictly Come Dancing & Dancing with the Stars

"Brilliant book. Highly motivational and altered my entire perspective around training and eating habits"
Dr Amalia Annaradnam
GP, Specialist in bio-identical hormones

"This is a great book, Dan really knows his stuff. I've learnt new techniques, exercises and practices to tailor my lifestyle for success"
James Redmond
Actor, Comedian and lanky streak of bacon

"Dan's training becomes a lifestyle that makes you stronger both physically and mentally."
Ian Camfield
Radio X Presenter

"Inspirational and practical. A dynamic manual for change."
David Lawson
Company Director and Author of '20 Minutes to Master Your Psychic Potential'

Legal Disclaimer

The publisher and the author make no representations or warranties with respect to the accuracy or completeness of the contents of this work and specifically disclaim all warranties including, without limitation, warranties for a particular purpose. No warranty may be created or extended by sales or promotional materials. The advice and strategies contained herein may not be suitable for every situation.

Neither the publisher nor the author shall be liable for damages arising herewith. The fact that an organization or website is referred to in this work as a citation and/or as a potential source of further information does not mean that the author or the publisher endorses the information the organization or website may provide or recommendations it may make.

Further, readers should be aware that websites listed in this work may have changed or disappeared between when this work was written and when it is read.

Acknowledgments

I have had many mentors, teachers & guides throughout my career. Each one provided a unique sprinkle of stardust to my current knowledge & understanding of the human body.

All roads have lead to this point.

Some helped shape me as a person & mold my character, others helped shape my business & some influenced my approach to health & my role within society.

However, they are all related.

I am thankful to you all. There are too many of you to mention individually. You know who you are & I am truly grateful for what you shared with me.

A special thank-you for total inspiration & growth acceleration:

- For clarity of thought & how to improve my focus through control of my mind, I thank Charles Haarnel.

- For an endless supply of knowledge for fat loss, strength & sporting performance, I thank Charles Poliquin.

- For helping me understand & integrate greater balance into my life through physical-mental-emotional-spiritual well-being, I thank Paul Chek.

- For providing structure & support for the creation of this book I thank Daniel Priestley & his KPI method.

- For help with images big thanks to Sergio Galvan Photography

For helping edit this document, I give special thanks to Emma, who not only supports & encourages my every effort, but also inspires me to be a better, happier man.

For support & never ending guidance, I thank my family *especially my Dad & Gary*, you are always there to help me in every way you can. You are the solid base on which I build my life.

In particular, my Mum, who is a rock. You are the stimulus to my success & a constant source of unconditional love, support & guidance. You teach me so much every day.

I can never be grateful enough.

I wholeheartedly thank you all.

Contents

Health**Wealth**

Feel Like A Billion Dollars
Every Day Of The Week

To be Optimal means to be the Best or most Favourable. As most people these days are so busy they usually find themselves in a sub-optimal state.

Their health & / or their wealth may suffer at some point or at the same time.

If you ever experience prolonged bouts of fatigue or tiredness, illness that won't clear up or any state where you do not feel at your best then you are not experiencing yourself at optimal.

HealthWealth was created to get you into your optimal state of being as quickly as possible & keep you there.

The quickest route from A to B is a straight line. What follows are the quickest routes to optimal health & performance. The roots of which, by natural osmosis, influence every area of your life.

The principles that I am about to place before you, once applied, will deliver you into an optimal state of being. The system as a whole is delivered through four solutions: Lifestyle, Exercise, Nutrition & Supplementation.

I will now introduce you to the system…

"You can't solve a problem on the same level it was created. You have to rise above it to the next level"

– Albert Einstein.

Foreword From The Author

I believe that if you live your life a certain way that you can achieve an optimal state of being.

If you eat a certain way, if you sleep a certain way, if you move a certain way, if you apply certain principles in a specific way that you slowly but surely bring yourself toward your personal best.

Once you achieve this state of being the circumstances of your life & the way in which you perceive them will be optimal & you will be happier as a result...

- Daniel Grant, London, 2015

Introduction to Optimalism™:

Doctrine: *is a codification of beliefs or a body of teachings or instructions, taught principles or positions, as the essence of teachings in a given branch of knowledge or belief system.*

Often doctrine specifically suggests a body of religious principles as it is proclaimed by a church, but not necessarily; doctrine is also used to refer to a principle of law, in the common law traditions, established through a history of past decisions, such as the doctrine of <u>self-defence</u>.

In some organisations, doctrine is simply defined as "that which is taught", in other words the basis for institutional teaching of its personnel internal ways of doing business.

This Book As A Doctrine…

The longevity of your success relies heavily on the performance of critical elements of your being.

I have been a personal health & fitness consultant for over 15 years & we could focus solely on physical training to bring about a breakthrough in that area of your life. There are many books on this subject alone.

However I know that peak physical fitness & optimal health (Optimalism) relies on so much more than just that one element.

It is a universal fact that when a human being aligns themselves with a higher principle, or set of higher principles, they become mighty. These principles are not essentially for self-gain or riches or material pleasure, although they could at some points in the process appear that way.

They are for the greater good of everyone on the planet. As when you are full of health & vitality you are able to give & keep giving of yourself.

In a similar way that religious beliefs offer a moral code by which to live, Optimalism offers a code of which to live by that makes optimal living a reality.

The way of living that I propose brings about your optimal state - in mind, body & spirit. As you refine the principles of Optimalism to your life, you will feel stronger – physically, mentally & emotionally.

I provide within this book a doctrine of health & fitness. A set of specific principles that once followed stimulates a higher state of being on a mental, physical & emotional plane.

Through attaining this state you are granted the power to 'keep-going'… the ability to remain optimistic through all circumstances… through which the world is your oyster & nothing can ever stand in your way.

I suggest that the more optimal your state of health & fitness – physically, mentally & emotionally, the more divine your life will appear to you & others… The more you will be able to serve yourself & others around you.

What Is Optimalism…

Optimalism is the combined meaning of the following words:

Optimum
Best; most likely to bring success or advantage.

Optimism
The quality of being full of hope & emphasising the good parts of a situation, or a belief that something good will happen.

Optimise
To make something as good as possible.

Optimist
Someone who always believes that good things will happen.

Optimal
Best or most favourable.

'What Optimalism Means To Me...
A set of principles to live by that produce an optimal state of being. Follow these principles & you gain access to an optimal life'

Further Developments...

*To be **optimistic** is when one expects the best possible outcome from any given situation.*

To remain optimistic in life is a skill that can be practiced, honed & mastered.

This is certainly a vital skill & studies have proven that those who remain optimistic are less susceptible to illness & disease.

Research has emerged showing the relationships between several psychological constructs & health. Optimism is one of these concepts, & has been shown to explain between 5–10% of the variation in the likelihood of developing some health conditions, notably including cardiovascular disease, stroke, & depression.

Laura Kubzansky Ph.D., M.P.H. is Associate Professor of Social and Behavioral Sciences & Director of the Society and Health Psychophysiology Laboratory, is at the forefront of such research.

In a 2007 study that followed more than 6,000 men & women aged 25 to 74 for 20 years, for example, she found that emotional vitality— a sense of enthusiasm, of hopefulness, of engagement in life, & the ability to face life's stresses with emotional balance—appears to reduce the risk of coronary heart disease. The protective effect was distinct & measurable, even when taking into account such wholesome behaviours as not smoking & regular exercise.

Among dozens of published papers, Kubzansky has shown that children who are able to stay focused on a task & have a more positive outlook at age 7, report better general health & fewer illnesses 30 years later. She has found that optimism cuts the risk of coronary heart disease by half.

Philosophy...

This is one example of a principle that can dramatically affect your life. Remaining Optimistic or holding an optimistic outlook. So many do not take advantage of this simple approach. This is where my philosophy of Optimalism comes to the forefront.

To go one step further, *William Godwin, English journalist, political philosopher & novelist hoped that society would eventually reach the state where calm reason would replace all violence & force, that mind could eventually make matter subservient to it, & that intelligence could discover the secret of immortality.*

Maybe this is optimism at its highest point? But how do you propose the human race could reach for this godly state? I suggest a higher state of experience can be achieved through diligent practice of specific principles that enhance a person's well-being.

There is little argument that specific movements build the strength & size of the correlating / working muscles.

I suggest that specific principles could also be applied to build a person's mental & emotional well-being. The combined set of principles could then bring about a quantum leap of a person's level of health & fitness. Profoundly affecting one's life for the better.

Elusive Info...

The specific practices required to grow in the above mentioned areas appear to be elusive to the average individual. Only those at the top of their game appear to be in possession of such priceless information.

For instance Michael Jordan, arguably the greatest basketball player of all time, a baseball pro, an entrepreneur, celebrity, clothing range owner, collaborator with Nike, retired & made a successful comeback twice! Both times breaking records for games & points scored. Not to mention breaking TV viewing records at the point of return from his first retirement. Olympic athlete & gold medalist, businessperson & actor. The first NBA star to become a billionaire.

Even if you know very little about Michael Jordan you will have heard his name & you certainly know this, he is a success. He certainly lives through the principles that bring success.

Michael possessed talent but he also applied himself in a very specific way that enabled his talent to experience its full potential. He lives by principles throughout his life that offer him the greatest chance of success in everything he does.

Ghandi is an example from another end of the spectrum. He held high principles in relation to human existence. He believed in freedom & equality for everyone. Gandhi led India to independence & inspired movements for civil rights & freedom across the world. He did this through non-violent demonstrations & holding an unbreakable set of principles.

The power is already inherent within the principle. Once a person aligns their thoughts, words & actions with a principle they become infinitely stronger. When a group forges this bond they become unstoppable.

Ghandi organically grew a peaceful-army from a nation, based on principle. The power of the principle (which can be accessed by anyone) is held within the principle.

It gives a person purpose & once aligned with the requirement of the principle, some of the decisions a person will be required to make from day-to-day will automatically be answered by what the principle dictates. This takes away the potential of being at the volatile whim of our fluctuating mind & emotions.

Your Body Is A Temple...

Religion provides a moral code to live by. Optimalism that I speak of here, provides a life code. Just like when a religious person makes regular visits to their place of worship, you will grow a practice of regular visits to yours… knowing that your body is in fact a temple!

As you live these principles day-in, day-out, your power will grow. I propose that the highest principles that you can live by in this day & age are those that which lead you to optimal health & fitness.

You could choose to hold religious or doctrine like beliefs around your health & fitness that stimulate optimal states of being - physically, mentally & emotionally.

This is not to say that you should immediately become a narcissistic, self-obsessed, egomaniac! But on the contrary become more aware of everything & everyone around you & how you can help them or the situation & yourself.

If at any moment in your life you are too ill to care for another in time of need, or not in a place financially to help another in time of need, or not confident enough in the aesthetics of your body to boost another's self-esteem – then I suggest that you are not in an optimal state.

That is why I invite you to practice 'Optimalism' in your life.

You may not apply all of the principles simultaneously but they provide you with a foundation to base your thoughts, words & actions around – in order to reach & remain in optimal state.

When you are in an optimal state of being you are at your personal best.

When you are in an optimal state of being you are a power to be reckoned with.

When you are in an optimal state of being you are able to give & keep giving of yourself.

When you are in an optimal state of being you can be of the most service to yourself & others...

Now I ask you what is more religious than that?

Welcome to a new type of religion, welcome to *Optimalism*.

A Little About The Author...

My name is Daniel Grant & I am a body-shaping expert with over fifteen years of experience as a personal health & fitness consultant.

There comes a point in a motivated, successful *professional's* life when he or she has everything—except perhaps *perfect* health & physical fitness. I close the gap between these two fundamentals.

When people ask me what I do for a living, I say, "I help people reach & remain at their personal best."

I've worked diligently over the past 17 years to grow my body, my knowledge & my business to a point where I can offer real insight & guidance to those who wish to improve their well-being without wasting time.

I coach & physically train high-flying, high achieving individuals & teams to reach & remain at their personal best. I love what I do, as I get to see, experience & be part of phenomenal success stories. I have seen that personal & financial success can be influenced directly by your well-being – I have seen this many times over.

For many years now I have been fully booked, accepting business through referral by appointment only. I've also co-developed two iPhone apps that put personal training in your pocket.

If you're a highflier who works crazy hours, thrives on making strong business decisions & are perhaps consumed by your business—but still want to have the benefits of a healthy, strong body—I am your guy.

When you couple a busy life with a busy mind, your body might suffer. A weak body leads to a weak mind.

I want to help you turn that sad equation into busy life, busy mind & vital body. To make this a reality, I developed a system that can work for you.

A Lifestyle...

This book contains a number of principles to live by. It is essentially a four-step guide that offers a quick fix to many health & fitness challenges—but at the same time it's a long-term solution to your overall health & fitness goals. It is not a diet, or an exercise program - It is a lifestyle.

I've spent many hours & put in lots of hard work with my clients & my own body over the years to hone & refine the system that you find within this book. It is the culmination of many lectures, study, listening, watching, attempting, correcting, improving, trial & errors to finally arrive at the concepts that actually work.

I have tried & tested all of the principles within this book. Some may appear very subtle but all of them deliver long-term positive improvement to your well-being & success.

When you follow my guidance, you will completely change the way your body looks & feels for the better—permanently!

I focus on the concept of duality in everything I do & it's a theme that pervades this book—positive / negative, muscle / fat, light / dark & so on.

If you see any imbalance in your life right now, then it's just a matter of time before a real physical or mental problem arises.

This book offers you many highly effective techniques for properly balancing your health & wellness.

I believe you were born to be great in every way. When you have a plan in motion carrying you toward that birthright, you are already half way to winning the battle.

From making the right lifestyle adjustments, to exercising correctly, to focusing on the best nutrition & supplementation options—I'll cover the principles that will help you build a strong, effortlessly powerful body.

I will provide you principles that you can live by that ensure you reach & remain at optimum.

This book will help you answer the question, "How can I strike the right balance that leads to optimum health & wellness while living a busy successful life?"

By focusing on the four key sections of Lifestyle, Exercise, Nutrition, Supplementation, I will get you to the point where being strong & healthy in body & mind, as well as being a super achiever is who you are.

- Daniel Grant

...Let's begin.

Solution 1: Lifestyle

Chapter 1: Health God

To keep the body in good health is a duty, otherwise we shall not be able to keep our mind strong and clear.

—Buddha

Stumbling blocks exist on every person's path to Optimalism. You have discovered a positive guide that will help you navigate these pitfalls, minimise mistakes & get you to your optimal state as quickly as possible.

You may have incredible success in within your area of expertise or with your business, but do you have the body to match? Does your body (& mind) have equal longevity?

Imagine getting ill & never reaching your true potential. It's likely that not many people will remind you that your body cannot keep up with your mind if you do not plan for it.

The Drive for Physical Perfection

There is nothing more natural than wanting to look & feel great. Having a body that resembles that of a Greek god or Goddess is a common desire. There's nothing wrong with wanting the best; after all, it's in your nature.

Feeling strong, confident & able is in your blood. Successful entrepreneurs have a natural drive for perfection & this applies to your physical state too.

Duality is present within everything & it's a theme that pervades this book. If you can already see or feel an imbalance, then there is most definitely an underlying problem.

This book offers a lot of techniques to properly balance your health & wellness.

I believe you were born to be great. You're likely already achieving this within your work life—now is the time to achieve this level of greatness with your body.

As soon as you have a plan for how & when you are heading toward that goal, you are already halfway to achieving it.

It's hard work achieving peak physical fitness, but with the right road map, anyone can get there.

With a special map, you can get there in half the time. This book is your map!

Lifestyle & the Troops

Do you live a general lifestyle, or are you the general of your life?

Most people are on autopilot; they lead reactive instead of proactive lives.

Understanding cause & effect is the root of constant success. I'll bet that you created the successes you have already achieved from conscious choices about who you wanted to be at specific moments in your life. A strong business decision that lead to growth & success.

The root of success is connected to your mind, the way you think about your life & how you apply your behaviors to it. Your thoughts, words & actions determine the outcome.

Your new challenge is to answer this question: What thoughts, words & actions do I need to take in order to achieve optimal health & fitness?

Think about this question for a moment – 'Are there specific principles that you can live by that will ensure your long-term success in every area of your life?'

If you carry on doing what you have been doing, you will keep on getting what you have been getting! Not much will change. That is why many of the things I recommend in this book are *outside of mainstream habit.*

You may need to try on a new approach or two in order to stimulate a different result.

Mainstream people do not march to their own tune - they follow the masses. Maybe you already march to your own tune? In which case I congratulate you, especially if you are happy with your success.

It is human nature to repeat old mistakes & to accept the reality that you are given. But you have a choice. With your courage & intelligence, you can wade through the parameters that lead people to be average & instead come out exceptional in *everything* you do.

Do you want more? How badly do you want it?

To achieve total success in mind & body, you have to master the four pillars of Optimalism:

1. *Lifestyle*—the choices you make on a day-to-day basis
2. *Exercise*—how you move & train your body
3. *Nutrition*—your food & beverage choices
4. *Supplementation*—how you support all your efforts.

Motivation over Time

What has stopped you from becoming outrageously fit in the past?

I bet one of your answers is time, right? You cannot stockpile health for long-term benefits. You must consistently & regularly repeat specific principles in order to maintain or develop your level of health & fitness.

If you don't use it – you lose it! Fact.

I'd bet that whenever you've tried to reach a new level of fitness (or health) in the past, you've always had the experience that something is missing. You may have thought that it was just time – you simply need more time in order to get better results.

Instead, consider that it could be approach & it could be the combination of techniques that you are applying that have left you with the feeling of lack.

What would benefit you the most is a way to apply yourself—mentally, physically & emotionally—to train your body to get the results you desire in half the time.

Learning about daily habits, food choices, training systems & supplementation can increase your rate of success.

This system will save you time by piecing each area together in a highly effective manner that works fast once you combine all of the elements.

Were the diets, exercises & systems you tried before not quite right for you? This one can be a perfect fit. Why? Because you will personalise each area to perfectly suit you & your requirements.

Mastering each principle within the system of Optimalism ensures that you accept these changes & make them new habits, so that they continue in your life, long after you have achieved your initial goals - you can live by these principles.

I know because I once tried everything & anything to achieve a healthy body; nothing ever seemed to work for long. I know how frustrating it can be.

I have been discovering & testing what actually works for many years now. This means that the principles within this book have been carefully formulated over many years.

You will be able to record the when, where & how as part of this program. To work, the principles need to become part of your daily schedule – your lifestyle.

You already know that time matters. The system will help you focus on the areas in your life where you need more balance, because right now there may be none or a clear imbalance?

Principle Exercise 1
Direct Your Day

Every moment of it. Write down a brief overview of a twenty-four hour period.

Include planned work hours & business meetings, foreseeable social events, time with family, children or loved ones, projected sleep times, etc.

This should take no more than ten minutes.

Now create a timeline for a week. Use an empty diary for example. This already has the hours, days & months set out for you to simply input your data.

Can you spot any clear imbalances?

Maybe you spend seventy hours at your desk every week.

When you see it this way, you may rethink how your life is passing day-by-day.

Is this what you want to be doing?

Is this what you need to be doing to live the life you desire?

Spending seventy hours sitting at a desk is not healthy. You don't need me to tell you that. Maybe you clearly see that you spend only 2 hours of quality time per week with the people you love? This is another form of imbalance.

It's just a matter of time before a real problem arises.

Time doesn't appear to go far when your lifestyle is hectic.

Begin to think about reallocating the hours in your day according to a new, balanced schedule that you deliberately choose.

After working diligently on a business a person can become consumed by it. I believe this may be a requirement of extreme success but unless that person pulls back a little at some point to re-balance their life, all could be lost & they will likely discover in the end that it was not worth it!

So balancing your day means a number of things:

1) *To balance the activities throughout your day, so that you are not doing 1 specific thing obsessively, day in - day out.*

2) *To highlight long-term imbalance like not seeing loved ones for weeks on end.*

3) *Something previously unforeseen may become clear to you. Looking at your entire week this way can bring to your attention situations in your life that where hidden from immediate view.*

Some Quick & Simple Solutions to Apply to A Hectic Day:

1) Organise a standing desk.
Studies prove that a standing desk results in a higher work output.

One study from Knight and Baer within the journal Social Psychological and Personality Science hypothesised that standing work spaces produced more ideas, greater collaboration & higher signs of engagement. [1]

---

1 Published online before print June 12, 2014, doi:10.1177/1948550614538463Social Psychological and Personality Science June 12, 20141948550614538463

2) Stand up & walk around for ten minutes of every one and half hours.

Like the flow of night & day as a cycle, called circadian rhythm, there are many cycles that operate throughout your day. Another important cycle is your ultradian rhythm. This is any biological process that displays oscillation of less than 24 hours. I specifically bring your attention to the 90-120 minute brain wave frequency cycle that occurs when we are both awake & asleep. [2]

Psychophysiologist Peretz Lavie demonstrated within his study of young adults that we get exceptionally sleepy at two times per day: 4:30pm & 11:30pm. But in the morning we get sleepy every 90 minutes. These 90-minute cycles are our ultradian rhythms, which define when we're naturally feeling awake & productive. You will perform better in between your periods of drowsiness.

- Set a timer on your phone & follow it. Numerous studies also show that having a ten-minute walk or break within this 90 minute period increases work output. It's about creating a balance or contrast of intensity. The active recovery period allows for recharge & another period of higher intensity to follow.

3) Schedule your day to different environments.

Schedule your day to make phone calls, work on your phone or laptop outside or in a quiet standing space to get you off your butt & on your feet more.

Altering your environment throughout your day has shown to increase dopamine secretion. Dopamine is a hormone & neurotransmitter that is essential for optimal function of your brain & body. It is important for nerve cell signaling in your brain (for

---

2 Ultradian Rhythms in Prolonged Human Performance, Peretz Lavie, Jacob Zomer, and Daniel Gopher, Institute of Technology, Haifa, Israel

instance to feel fully awake or alert) & for the controlled release of other hormones in your body.[3]

Alter your route to the office or home, make your calls in different areas of your home, office or simply select a different place to where you usually are. If you happen to work on your laptop, sit in a different place each time you start a timed work period.

Tailor the above suggestions to best suit your environment.

Main point right now is to make the change, soon after you will begin to benefit from these simple steps.

---

3 http://www.bps.org.uk/news/study-questions-dopamines-part-adhd

Principle 1:
I Control The Direction Of My Day.

Highlight the areas of your life that are out of balance.
Improve at least one imbalance this coming week.

Complete this exercise for the coming weeks.
Select one imbalance-correction goal every week.

When you apply the suggestions made above they will eventually become part of who you are! I make this statement because you are a high achiever; by picking up this book you have demonstrated that you are looking for an even better way to do things.

The reason this is the first principle is that it has you take an overview
look at your life. You get to adjust anything that is immediately & obviously out of balance.

As soon as you make an adjustment you can benefit from it.

Each week you'll be able to factor in more balance as the last adjustment you made has become part of your life, & it did so easily because it made your day flow more smoothly – it made your life easier or made you happier.

Once you establish greater balance, you have made the first step toward Optimalisation.

Before you take a look at your daily diary, or even your week, set the tone & make the statement "I Control The Direction Of My Day" – then begin organising.

This is the first principle to apply to your life if you havn't already.

The Dangers of Stress Unleashed

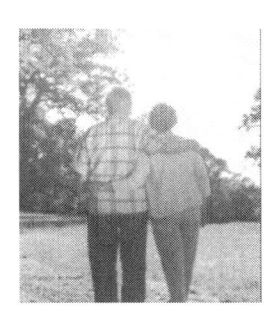

Let me make this clear from day one—unmanaged day-to-day stress is the worst thing that can happen to your health. It is one of the largest & most difficult stumbling blocks to get over.

Stress is a moment-by-moment part of modern day life. For many entrepreneurs, it's a way of life. It becomes a habit that won't go away.

We experience an estimated one hundred times greater stress level than our grandparents.

There are two distinctions to make about stress:

1) Positive Stress.
Some stress brings about positive experiences. For example, studies show that people who are happy with their stressful jobs have similar brain activity to people ten years younger.

Dr. Lachman is one of the principal investigators for what could be considered the Manhattan Project of middle age, an <u>enormous study</u> titled Midlife in the United States, or Midus.

Everyone in the study who regularly did more to challenge their brains — reading, writing, attending lectures or completing word puzzles — did better on fluid intelligence tests than their counterparts who did less.

And those with the fewest years of schooling showed the largest benefits. Middle-age subjects who had left school early but began working on keeping their minds sharp had substantially better memory & faster calculating skills than those who did not. They responded as well as people up to 10 years younger. In fact, their scores were comparable to college graduates.

Stress from leadership is healthy—not unhealthy.

Another example of positive stress is a deadline that requires you to complete a piece of wok. Once the task is completed you, have created something of value that brings you happiness. However, reaching that goal involved stress.

This is called Eustress. This term was originally explored in a stress model by Richard Lazarus. It is the positive cognitive response to stress that is healthy, or gives one a feeling of fulfilment or other positive feelings. This term was created as a subgroup of stress to differentiate the wide variety of stressors & manifestations of stress.

Remember that even too much positive stress can pull you out of balance leaving your system drained. You must keep an eye on this. More importantly your immediate attention should be on taking care of more damaging stress…

2) Negative Stress.
This type of stress usually comes from not being in control of an outcome. When you try your best to have a situation work out in your favor, but it doesn't, the end result is stress, leading to more stress.

There are many other inlets of stress in to your body on a day-to-day basis. Noise, environmental, quality of food (or lack of), emotional, relationship, financial, workload… the list goes on.

Stress is unavoidable. The real trick is how best to deal with it.
I am going to help you with that as you read on.

This section of the book deals with negative stress.

Because positive stress is, as it suggests, positive, be happy & accept it into your life, if you have not done so already.

There are ways to master the stress that appears to be out of your control—negative stress.

Stressing the Matter...

- *Checking for danger is a stress response.* It may be human nature to think of safety & survival often, but the chances of you being attacked by a lion walking down Oxford Street or Rodeo Drive are zero. However, be careful when crossing the street!

- *Your body overreacts to any stress response.* You can reduce your stress levels when you are clear on three criteria: 1) Know where you are right now, physically & mentally. 2) Take responsibility for where you are going from this point. 3) Have a plan of how to get to where you want to go. Once you have these three criteria handled you will reduce your day-to-day anxiety & stress levels. It is subtle but useful. Think of the story about the final piece of straw that broke the camels back! It wasn't that one tiny piece of straw but the accumulation of stress that finally overpowered the animal.

- *Stress from your family.* This stress tends to be held close to your heart. If you think about an argument with, or the loss of, a family member, it is like a firecracker going off in your head & chest. Learning to deal with this is important.

- *Direct worry from actual situations—***illness, bills & business.** To handle your stresses, know exactly where they come from & how to manage them.

- **Stress from money.** This does not benefit you in any way. Evaluate your feelings on money & the stress that surrounds you because of it. This book introduces techniques to handle this.

- **Observe & acknowledge your personal stress level.** Think about what you can do to improve it? Solving stress-related issues can help. Use Principle 1 to help you highlight where your main source(s) of stress originate. Get to the root & deal with it ASAP.

- **Analyse & solve your problems.** Meet stress head on; understand it & then ground yourself in adequate solutions for it. Again, I provide useful techniques & solutions later on.

- **Stress from your own thoughts.** If a stressful thought has no benefit for you, drop it. Directly replace negative thoughts with positive ones. Replacement is the only way to achieve this. A positive & negative thought cannot occupy your head at the same time. It's one or the other. You choose.

- **Know your character as though it were someone who lived outside of you.** Immerse yourself in who you are & if necessary tweak any negative characteristics. This must be done over time & has no short-term method or shortcut of achieving the change. It is honesty toward yourself & taking responsibility for what happens in your life. How you think, speak & move affects your life – how can you affect every situation in a way that is positive for you? Something for you to practice – forever.

Do not excuse away judgmental thoughts, because they can be stressful. Measure the impact that all this stress has on your life.

Much of something brings more. If you worry all the time, more worry will come of it. If you are positive all the time, that breeds a positive outlook.

Be aware of who you are & how you think. It affects your stress levels. Don't deny your emotions. They make you who you are. Let them flow & acknowledge them. Understanding them is the key to continuous success.

The Language of Your Body

You communicate most with your body language. In fact, 55 percent of your communicate is through your body language. The rest comes from your tone of voice (38 percent) & choice of words (7 percent). This sub-communication is a powerful force that you can tap into.

In the 1960s Dr. Albert Mehrabian (UCLA) ran experiments that resulted in this understanding of communication & it is now an important element in kinesics.

Body language & tone of voice are far more important than the words you choose.

- *Refine your body language & tone of voice to increase the power of your communication.* Confident people do this naturally. They talk louder & deeper, hold their chest & heads up & smile. Maybe you could make a small improvement in this area?

- *How do women know when a man is lying?* A lot of this can be chalked up to a heightened sense of body language, which is also linked to peripheral vision. Women use more of their peripheral vision than men. True feelings are easier to spot if you focus on body language.

- ***Men use tunnel vision,*** which is why they need to turn their whole head when they check out a woman as they walk past. Women don't have to turn their heads—they make more use of their peripheral vision. Open up your vision to become more aware of your surroundings at all time – a good practice to adopt for both men & women.

- ***Compare someone you know who is fit with someone you know who is unfit.*** The unfit person likely won't seem as confident or dynamic as the fit person. What you think of yourself matters—how do you feel about your current appearance? Whatever your current physical state, it's time to dial-up the positivity a notch or two…We'll deal with how you look as we progress through this book.

- ***Own the space you are in.*** Wherever you are, be there—not miles away, somewhere in your head. Begin by simply stating in your mind that you have control over your space. This will energise you & you'll instantly begin to hold a confident body position.

- ***Stand still in your space.*** Take a deep breath in & let it out slowly. Imagine you have achieved everything you desire. Put yourself there; it removes your stress.

Once you have this mind-set, notice how you carry yourself. Do people treat you differently? Of course they will.

Everyone is drawn to confident, successful people. It is not how high you climb, but how you climb that truly matters.

Live your life in a certain way & you can enjoy every single moment. It really is a choice.

This is about your health—potentially *the* most crucial element in your life. If you do not have your health then you cannot experience anything freely. Evaluate how you present yourself to the world & adjust it for the better.

Become more aware of how you hold your body when you have conversations. Be more aware of your posture as you sit at your desk. Be more aware of your body & how you control each movement of every day.

Managing your body movements & increasing your body awareness will reduce your stress levels & increase positive outcomes in your life.

There are always improvements you can make-that is one of the never-ending beauties of life.

Attraction Pays Big

Being attractive can be important. Attractive people emanate something special that draws others toward them. When you are at optimal health, your powers of attraction go through the roof.

- ***When you are healthy, you are capable.*** You have more stamina & can get things done. Achieving greater health will make you stand out from 80 percent of the crowd & increase your chance of success in business.

- ***You have more innate energy.*** You can outperform people & get better "life" conversions. Meaning that your circumstances are optimal or more to your liking. The gym, bedroom, sports field & boardroom—they all convert to happiness more effectively when you apply more energy. What you put in is what you get out.

- ***Reproductive potential.*** Your options improve & your lifespan increases when you are healthy. This is extremely attractive. Truly healthy adults usually have healthy kids & they are able to stand the external challenges that wear down the human body. Through this you increase your chances of finding a quality partner to share your life with. Or, if the single life is your game, you increase the quality of your options the healthier you are. When you are satisfied with your personal life this has positive affects across your business life & well-being.

- ***When you kiss someone you can taste how healthy he or she are.*** Weird, but true! Our brains test for health during saliva exchange. This can affect whom you end up with or who chooses to end up with you. This points to increasing your chances of you & a suitable mate finding each other. The happier you are at home the more likely you can focus on your business more effectively & your health can flourish.

- ***Better sex life.*** Being healthy increases how attractive you are. The more attractive you are, the better your sex life is. This is true for two reasons. 1) You feel better about yourself & therefore exude confidence & sex appeal. 2) As you stand out from the crowd, others notice you & are attracted to you. On the flip side, this can be a major stress factor if you are 'over doing it in the dating department!'

- ***Health = Stamina = Attraction.*** Optimal health allows you to enjoy the freedom of more stamina— better performance in the boardroom, in the bedroom & on the sports field.

Chapter 2:
Lifestyle Stress Test

In times of great stress or adversity, it's always best to keep busy, to plough your anger and your energy into something positive.

—Lee Iacocca

Focus on unearthing all your secret stress reactions that cause you to behave the way you do, so that you can intervene. For example, you might hunch your shoulders, get defensive, or over focus on details. Become aware of how you tend to react to situations, so you can respond more effectively.

It is critical that you apply techniques to help you manage stress effectively.

It simply isn't healthy to live with sky-high stress levels day after day, year after year.

Is Stress Hitting You Hard?

Stress can hit you from so many sources —as part of your lifestyle, your exercise routine, your nutrition & the supplements you take (or your body could be stressed from insufficient nutrient intake).

They all interlink & feed off each other. Solving stress in one area can help you resolve stress in other areas of your life.

- *Lifestyle:* A full understanding of how your lifestyle impacts your stress levels is the key to understanding how to reapply the way you think & act.

- *Exercise:* Your exercise routine needs to be evaluated. Acknowledge what you have, or have not, been doing. Say it out loud! Do you exercise? The American College of Sports Medicine recommends that adults exercise for at least one hundred & fifty minutes every week. That's thirty minutes five times a week at a moderate intensity. What is moderate? 75 percent of your maximum heart rate. What is your maximum heart rate? 220 minus your age.

  Build a body that you are proud of. Do you in fact exercise too often? This can also prevent you from achieving great results. We'll refine the details around these concepts as you read on.

- *Nutrition:* Is your diet healthy? How do you know? Everyone has different ideas on what healthy is in relation to the food that you eat. Not many of us have time to wade through three hundred new diet fads. What you need is solid, science-based nutrition that is geared toward healing & invigorating the human body. I'll help you set this up for your unique requirements.

- *Supplementation:* Should you be taking supplements? Which brands, how often & why? You need to find out what the right information is so that you don't end up under- or over nourished & miss out on optimum health.

Gandhi always said, "Be the change you wish to see in the world."
It's time to be the change you wish to see in yourself.

If you want a fitter, firmer body, stronger immune system & sharper mind then now is the time to apply specific principles that bring that experience to life.

Get Rid of Belly Fat, Once & for All

Where does all this stress-related fat show up on your body? Let me tell you!

The basic story goes like this, the more stressed you are, the more fat your body stores to withstand that stress. The more fat, the more stress your body can handle.

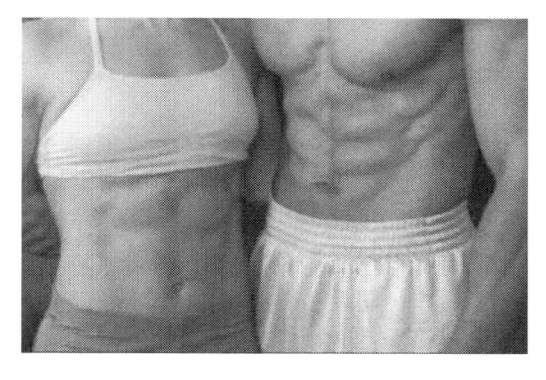

Stress can attract & hold fat to your body, even if you reduce your calorie intake.

You need to learn stress management in order to lose fat effectively.

If you're starting to grow a little muffin top belly listen up.

Toxicity in Your Body

- Toxicity causes obesity. Toxins can enter your body in many ways: through food, the environment, products you apply to your skin & so on. These can cause havoc. Healthy bodies excrete toxins, but unhealthy bodies allow illness & disease to take hold as a result of toxicity & the inability to get it out of the system. Amino acids, vitamins & minerals must be used wisely, along with exercise, nutrition & lifestyle management in order for your body to excrete toxins effectively.

- *A lot of toxins are stored within your body fat, away from your heart & internal organs.* As things get worse (you get more stressed & fatter), internal (visceral) fat can also build up around your internal organs. This is very unhealthy & in the long run extremely dangerous.

- In the first phase of fat build up, your body literally traps toxins within fat away from your organs in an attempt to keep you as healthy as possible. Those toxins cause a serious health risk if you attempt to lose fat too quickly. As what happens is the toxins are released from the stored fat in to your blood stream – this can make you feel extremely rough. You need to support & improve your detox pathways in order to get rid of it.

Stress in Your Body

- Stress happens. Only *you* can learn to control it by taking responsibility for your reactions. I was close to my grandparents & watched them get ill & eventually pass away. Then my mother was diagnosed with breast cancer. These experiences taught me what "real" stress feels like & gave me a totally different perspective about stress.

- Decrease stress; allow your emotions to happen. Reflect on & engage with your emotions. Do your best to understand them. Set goals & know where you are going. You are in control when you have a plan. Fight stress wherever it may hide. Your perception is the prime influencer over your stress levels. Alter your perception & you'll alter your stress levels—instantly.

Malnutrition in Your Body

- Malnutrition is shockingly common because modern food focuses on calories for energy instead of nutrient-rich foods. Lack of these nutrients leads to deficiencies that can trigger other problems in your body.

Think of your body as being made up of links like in a chain. Day-to-day life places stress on those links. Your body always breaks at the weakest link just like a chain.

Stress in whatever form causes the link to break. Inadequate nutrition may weaken every link in your body-chain.

Your mind, body & emotions govern these links & protect you against stress. The stronger you create each of the links within your system the more resilient you become to stress.

Stressed Hormones

Back to solving that belly fat problem. Where your body stores fat is related to your hormones.

Belly fat is where receptor sites for the stress hormone cortisol are commonly found.

When you are stressed out, cortisol causes you to gain fat in & around your belly. Therefore stress reduction is one of the main keys to losing belly fat. In fact, it is one of the missing elements in a lot of peoples approach to fat loss.

I use the same system Charles Poliquin, my mentor uses. The BioSignature Modulation process teaches you how to positively impact your belly fat.

Tips to Reduce Stress

- **Herbal adaptogens** have been used for centuries to decrease & manage stress. Most people will not be able to break their stress cycle & will require adaptogens. You must work with a skilled professional to determine your specific requirements. More about this later.

- **Over periods of prolonged stress,** *fat accumulates on your face.* Your chin & cheeks look fatter. If you reduce your stress, your face will eventually thin out again. Long-term stress management has dozens of other beneficial consequences.

- **What comes first for you:** *negative thoughts or negative body language?* **It is a chicken & egg scenario, but one that illustrates the point. Does an unhealthy lifestyle come first, or the disease? Negativity breads negativity, so changing to positive body language does, scientifically speaking, improve stress status. In Key Issues in Mental Health vol 174, Stress – The Brain-Body Connection, the editors point out that 'One of the most neglected realities in stress medicine is the profound dissociation between the psychological & the bodily stress response. In other words, a lot of people do not associate their symptoms (being mental or physical or both) with stress & therefore apply inadequate treatment plans.** [1]

---

1 https://books.google.co.uk/books?hl=en&lr=&id=AwvS1kzQuY8C&oi=fnd&pg=PP1&dq=body+language+and+stress&ots=a7it-WCPfB&sig=h5ZSKvHIZv97_CBWpW94riz25AM#v=onepage&q&f=false

- *Break your current cycle & apply a new, more positive outlook.* Re-train yourself to be even more effective. Be aware of your thoughts, words, body language & actions.

- *If your behavior does not match up with who you want to be, stop!* Take a deep breath, & then "pretend" to react how you would prefer to react. This will go a long way to correcting your negative behaviors. The saying, "Fake it till you make it" can be useful in some circumstances.

- *Change your tone of voice to impact your communication.* Deepen your voice, pushing down a little on your Adam's apple to create more bass. You can find your Adams apple near the center of your throat, when you swallow it will move up & down. This commanding tone will demand respect from others. Also it has been proven more effective to talk slower, even in high-pressure situations, much like how James Bond demands respect & talks slowly. For females think about the way in which Toni Braxton sings, lower depth than the average female singer. A deeper tone will also calm you & make you feel more grounded.

Happiness & enjoyment are directly related to how you process stress & how they trigger your hormones.

They have an inverse relationship.
The higher your negative stress, the less happy you are.
Or
The happier you are, the less stressed you will be.

To reduce belly fat, you must change your stress patterns. The first very simple step is to act positively & be aware of how you speak to others & to yourself (internal dialogue).

Your Perception Is Everthing

Stress can enter your life in any of the ways mentioned earlier. It impacts every part of you, which is why evaluating stress in your life is so crucial to this process.

Now that you have begun to highlight the areas that need work (Principle One), you can choose how your life runs from now on. Your perception of the world impacts how you react to every situation in your life.

Right now you may notice that you are stressed or on the flip side you may feel happy or even positively stressed as mentioned earlier – Eustress. Either way be aware that your perception in this very moment determines your experience.

Imagine for a moment wearing yellow-tinted glasses. Even though there are many colors in reality, all you'd see is yellow.

If you continued to wear these glasses 24 hours a day, after a while, you would begin to think that what you see is reality, everything is yellow — until you took those glasses off & all the richness of colour returned. That is what perception is like.

Think about changing the way you see the world. Do you give yourself freedom to see your character? Does your character suit your life goals or does it actually stand in the way of your true happiness or ultimate success? What, or who, you really want to be is all about your perception.

You don't need to experience life based on perceived stress. It's a waste of your time & energy. If your life is stressful, then take action to minimise that stress. Even if it is simply by altering your perception of your current circumstances.

Stop to smell the roses!

You don't always have to be in a rush, like most of the Western World.

There is a big difference between being busy, productive & successful, which, as mentioned, is good/positive stress. Negative stress prevents you from being your best. It will come up, so you need to notice when it happens.

By all means, be a high-energy hard working personality, but find your balance in the things that matter.

Adding in more de-stressors will stimulate growth, creativity & insight from within. It will also boost your productivity levels & prolong your life or at least the enjoyment of the fruits of your efforts.

Like a lion when it hunts, you want to reach a point where you can be still, patient & focused most of the time & then, when needed, use speed, timing & accuracy to pounce on your goals.

The first step is gaining control of your health & physical state. Then you will feel limitless in your abilities as a successful, able person, on top of your business accomplishments.

Charles Haarnel in his ever-popular book The Master Key System writes:

'Some men seem to attract success, power, wealth, attainment, with very little conscious effort; others conquer with great desires & ideals, Why is this so? Why should some men realize not at all?

The cause cannot be physical, else the most perfect men, physically, would be the most successful. The difference therefore must be mental – must be in the mind'.

Four Reasons Why Stress Dominates Your Life

If you were completely honest, you would probably admit that stress dominates your life. There are many subtle ways that it creeps in & seizes control. Anything can stress you out…if you allow it too.

Alternatively, you can repel stress like water running off a rain mac.

You are on your way to controlling your stress levels. Here is what you need to look out for in the coming days.

1: *What your parents & grandparents ate affects you today.*
You likely grew up eating things that you now know have almost no nutritional value! Maybe, you were '*treated*' to lots of sweets by your grandparents? Most grandparents like to smother their grand kids with things they like to eat. Most foods at the grocery store these days are high in calories, with low nutritional content – just like chocolate & sweets. Sweets, chocolate/candy, microwave meals, packaged & processed foods are the main culprits. On top of this the nutritional value of our food supply from '*good sources of food' like protein, fruit & vegetables* is also diminishing! Believe it.

2: *Your environment could be stressing you out.*
City life with its noise pollution & non-stop buzzing around you all the time takes its toll. It doesn't allow you to get proper rest when you sleep or experience one moment of peace in your day. Noise pollution, electromagnetic pollution (think Wi-Fi, computers & mobile phones) & chemical pollutants (think car/ truck fumes, chemical products on your skin & on

your food) are all playing their part in your overall level of health.

3: *Fumes, chemicals & toxins are all around you.*
They're found in your food, in your household cleaning products & even in the personal hygiene products you use. These days they are virtually impossible to avoid. Even if you live in the most remote parts of the world chemicals have been found that have never been used in that area. The chemicals are in our eco-system. They evaporate, enter our airwaves & rain down in other parts of the world. [1]

4: *Your body is 75 percent water.*
If you live in a big city like London, UK, the water from your tap is brimming with toxins, hormones & other chemicals. According to the latest study by Brunel University, water in the UK contains more than three hundred man-made chemicals.

This cannot be a good thing. If you constantly replace your body's water stores with impure water, it is bound to have affect on you mentally & physically. This may not show up right away, as the immediate effects of the toxins are not at a dangerous level from one glass of water or cup of tea.

However, could repeat exposure, year after year build up in your system & cause hormonal imbalances or disease within your body? I suggest you'd be much safer avoiding or cleansing your water as much as possible.

---

1 http://www.nrdc.org/health/

Principle Exercise 2
Subtle Stress Reduction

- *To combat noise pollution:*

Spend ten minutes in total silence each day. Do this at any time during
your day, but it will be especially effective before you go to bed. This will
help you wind down & get a better night sleep. Use earplugs, close your
eyes & breathe deeply.

- *For electromagnetic pollution:*

*Cut yourself off from laptops, mobiles/cell phones, TV & artificial
light for at least one hour before going to bed. Think about
candlelight & conversation! If you like to read before bed, turn the
lights down or only use just enough light so that you can read freely.
At bedtime, the less stimulation from light the better. Your skin
perceives light as a signal to get up – the opposite of what you want
as you are heading toward bedtime.*

*You could also invest in a product called Silvernet that blocks out
this pollution while you sleep.*

- *Environmental pollution:*

*Spend more time with nature. Go to the park; buy lots of plants.
Nature heals the effects of environmental pollution. Plants & trees
absorb pollution, saving you from breathing it in or absorbing it
into your body.*

- *Water pollution:*

*Only drink filtered or noncarbonated mineral water from glass
bottles.*

Drink between 1.5 & 3 liters of clean water every single day -
Equivalent to 6–12 cups

Studies show that drinking adequate amounts of fresh, clean water
daily decreases stress levels & belly fat. Who doesn't want that?

- ***Train but do not drain***

Build on your activity level by finding your challenge point, leaning
into it & resting afterward. Too much over activity can be stressful.

Get the balance that is right for you.

- ***Regular short interval breaks***

As explained earlier you will be more productive if you take regular
intervals while performing extended periods of focus —ten minutes
rest for every 90 minutes of focus. This has been proven to result in
greater productivity levels. Do less for more results.

- ***Regular vacation***

Take a "vacation" break every three months, for the same reason
mentioned above. Studies show that when you are fresh, you are
able to focus more effectively, you waste less time & get more done
in shorter periods of time. On top of which you will reduce your risk
of coronary heart disease!

A 9-year study following middle-aged men concluded that those
who did not take regular vacations suffered higher mortality rates,
particularly CHD.

Planning your work & rest schedules to create balance is the key.

If someone manages your diary for you get him or her to factor this
in, you will benefit in the long term for it.

Principle 2:
I Choose My Perception

Gain control of your inner stress levels by simply applying stress release points throughout your day, week, months & years.

Fail to plan these points into your life & you reduce your longevity & time at the top of your game. This is something that is directly in your control. It is also something that most of us neglect when focused on a long term project or goal.

Also remember that your perception is everything. It can be difficult to truly grasp this point for anyone who has never lost someone very close to his or her heart or suffered a near death experience. Whenever an experience of this sort occurs it totally alters ones perception of what is true stress & what can & can't be handled.

For instance, in a split second, you can realise that the death of a loved one is far more important than losing a large sum of money.

Manage your perspective everyday in every way & you go some way to managing your stress level & long-term level of health… & ultimately your happiness.

Apply the technique points on the previous page to reduce the amount of stress around you & notice the difference in your energy level, mood, productivity & well-being.

Stress the Truth

High stress levels cause disease & disorder. There are more doctors & greater access to medical health than ever before, but people are dying in droves & there is more illness than ever.

Take the rise of cancer & diabetes as a clear example.

We are members of the fattest, weakest humans to ever walk the earth. Who wants to be part of that statistic?

Perhaps it is because we live such high-stress lives.

Stress causes inflammation in your body. Your body makes more cholesterol when it is stressed. Your body will make more cholesterol to increase your resilience to stress. When inflammation is present it is common to see cholesterol levels rise.

Too much cholesterol is bad. Just the right amount of cholesterol is good.

Some cholesterol medications work by blocking a substance your body needs to make cholesterol. Statins may also help your body re-absorb cholesterol that has built up in plaques on your artery walls, preventing further blockage in your blood vessels and heart attacks.

So your body makes more cholesterol to deal with increasing stress levels, whatever the stress may be. But preventing your body from rushing to deal with the stress may not be the answer.

It's like stopping the firefighters on their way to the fire.

Taking cholesterol medication is a sign that your cholesterol is high. The best thing you can do is figure out why your cholesterol is high.

You need to understand where your inflammation is, where your stress comes from & why your body may be creating so much cholesterol.

Once you know what the cause is, work to reduce the cause or its effect on you. Then, with your doctor, keep an eye on your cholesterol levels. Optimalism's first 3 Principles will go some way to mitigating your stress response.

This should begin to reduce your stress levels & triggers. I will provide you with other means to support this reduction as you read on. A whole-istic approach is required, in that it is not one singular thing that is causes high cholesterol or high blood pressure for that matter.

When you apply all of the principles within this book, then with consent from your doctor, you may eventually reduce, or even completely eliminate meds. Deal with the cause & you automatically handle the effect.

James LaValle, clinical pharmacist, author & nutritionist put it very simply:
'Manage stress (cortisol) & you maximise performance'

- Stress is part of the condition of high blood pressure. The higher your stress levels, the more stress you place on your heart. Stress equals constriction, a narrowing of your blood vessels that, in turn, increases the pressure in your system because your heart has to pump harder to get blood around your body.

- Exercise helps lower stress by releasing the pressure & in turn improving blood pressure problems. When you check your blood pressure at home, make sure that the cuff is the correct size & that you take it in the morning when you first get out of bed, or false readings can occur. You can take your blood pressure several times a day to gain an accurate picture of your status.

- Many food cravings are a result of stress in your body. Increased consumption of sugar, caffeine & other stimulants is a sign that you are under stress. If you consume these types of food for too many days in a row too often, they can be dangerous & cause internal dysfunction—leading to even greater stress!

- Your body creates cortisol to improve the resistance of your cells to stress. High cortisol levels mean you are stressed in one way or another. Stress can come from any source & at any time.

- Cortisol can be a response to a fight-or-flight scenario. When you are faced with danger, your body creates adrenaline. Continued overstimulation results in high cortisol output.

- This response from your body can come from many sources. The root however is a prolonged imbalance - work/rest ratio, relationships, choice of food or drink, over exercising, sex life & the list goes on.

- Cortisol is meant to be high in the morning, waking you up when the sun hits your skin. It should begin moving away from its peak before midday. Then should continue to descend as the day goes on leading in to the evening. You need low cortisol levels at night to get proper rest. There are specific strategies to normalise cortisol curves that you can easily apply. We will talk more about these in a later section.

- *Learning to raise or lower your cortisol levels is one of the keys to gaining control of your overall health, body shape & performance levels.*

To better manage your stress levels, record in a journal or simply make a note in your phone where the stress is coming from. At least be precisely aware of when the stress hits your system & what caused it – then you can take definitive action.

If you notice patterns of stress-triggers, then it is time to do something about it. Decide to break those cycles & work on them. Identify the areas & apply improvement daily. If you cannot improve those situations after repeated efforts, it's time to reduce or eliminate where possible the root cause from your life.

The principles I suggest within this book will help you with this. Sometimes it is impossible to deny a stress. That is why I advise taking preventative measures before the stress-trigger. This way you manage your response before any potential negative situation has a chance to affect your system.

Exercise is a massive de-stressor. Movement gets your body working & brings better balance to your life. I'll help you better organise your training selection as you read on.

The clearer your perspective about each & every area of your life the more successful you will be. Constantly be the watchful gatekeeper at the peripheral of your body & mind.

Compare your stress levels to a friend's. Notice if you are more or less stressed than your friends & acquaintances. Are you able to remain the most relaxed person that you know?

As you read through this book you will gain a fresh perspective of your personal stress levels. Apply the principles within. Work on your breathing techniques & make de-stressing an essential part of your new lifestyle.

There will be a subtle ripple affect across your life. Like a pebble hitting the water, the ripple effects reach out across the water to the very edge. The same applies to your life. Improve one area & you will positively affect every other area.

Chapter 3:
Crush Your Stress

The more tranquil a man becomes, the greater is his success, his influence, his power for good. Calmness of mind is one of the beautiful jewels of wisdom.

—James Allen
Author, philosophical writer

Stress. You may be aware that it's a huge part of your life right now? Tell me, do you know anyone who is not stressed in one way or another? The only way you can let go of unhealthy areas of your lifestyle is to do exactly that—let go.

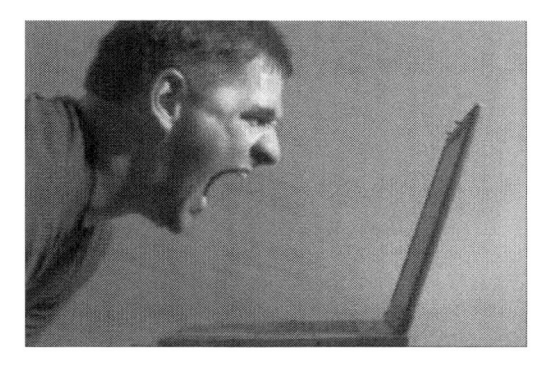

That's why you need to know how to lower your stress levels on a daily basis. Focus on these areas to reap the benefits of a reduced-stress lifestyle.

Work on small steps, day-by—day & subtly eliminate pockets of stress from your life.

Seize Control

- *Sleep properly for seven to nine hours a night on a minimum of four nights per week—every week.*

- Be **positive** every day in every way you can. When you notice stress rising, break out your positivity. The two cannot exist in the same space. If you struggle, try combining positivity with motion for an added boost—either motion in your mind, such as imagining the positive scenario, or physically get your body moving. Put on a big smile on your face, uncross your arms & legs & open up your body language. Your mind will follow.

- Do not open **mail** after eight pm, particularly business related - you must manage your stress levels effectively, especially at night. Mail must wait till the morning. If you truly want optimal health & fitness you must prioritise *You*. Everything else, including your business will eventually benefit from this shift. When you position all mail toward the beginning of your day it will help to normalise your cortisol levels giving you energy when you need it & the ability to wind down & recuperate at the perfect time.

- Swap **artificial** lights for candles by eight o'clock. This will reduce light exposure to your skin, which will help to naturally lower your cortisol levels & prepare you for sleep.

- Don't **eat** food that is high in sugar after four o'clock. Focus on vegetables & proteins. We'll delve into this in detail later on in the book.

- **Supplement** your diet where you see obvious deficiencies. For instance drink a green juice everyday if you know you do not eat enough green vegetables. Get tested to find out exactly what vitamins &

minerals you are lacking & also what foods may be aggravating your system. More about this later.

- **Blood tests** are an accurate way to determine exactly what your body lacks. I offer a system for testing nutritional deficiencies & then apply methods to improve the identified area(s). Clients who use my blood-testing procedure experience dramatic improvements to their health & fitness levels within a matter of weeks.

- Life is about **balance**. Where is your life out of balance? You should have a good idea about this from the first principle at the start of this book.

- Computers act as **stimulants**, so apply rules to balance your use of electronics. These can fatigue you & cause you untold stress. Stop using them by eight o'clock—at the latest—every night. This will give you a better chance of sleeping well, lowering body fat, reducing your stress levels & gaining muscle. Try getting to sleep earlier so you can wake earlier, get on with business & not be exhausted by midday!

- Get the right amount of **sex**—not too much & not too little. Studies show that the ideal amount in terms of health is between three times per week & once a day. Your health status will determine what is best for you. Use trial & error to see what leaves at your best. Enjoy!

- Notice how you **talk** to others & to yourself. According to Brian Tracy "Self-esteem is the relationship you have with yourself," Brian Tracy is an entrepreneur, public speaker & author of several books about personal & professional development.

- Practice guided **meditation**. You can also call this "reflection time." I'll help you set this up later in the book.

- Cut out obvious harmful **substances** to your body. Cut back or quit smoking, alcohol consumption, energy drinks, caffeine & so on. Handle this area right now. Again I will provide you guidelines around what I have found & what the current research says about consumption of these substances as you read on.

Enemy Number One

It's true. Stress is enemy number one for your body, mind & spirit.

According to a long-term population study,[1] stress is a serious risk factor for mortality rates. Highly stressed people die sooner than people who experience less stress.

People who are calmer & less stressed have also been found to live longer, happier lives. Mindfulness-based stress reduction lowers blood pressure, according to the American Psychosomatic Society.[2]

Stress has to be replaced with something else. I suggest you replace it with a contemplative thought that will, in turn, stimulate good health, positivity & a longer life.

---

1 Carolyn Aldwin, Nuoo-Ting Molitor, "Do Stress Trajectories Predict Mortality in Older Men? Longitudinal Findings from the VA Normative Aging Study," *Journal of Aging Research*, http://www.hindawi.com/journals/jar/2011/896109/.

2 "Mindfullness-based Stress Reduction Helps Lower Blood Pressure Study Finds," http://www.sciencedaily.com/releases/2013/10/131015094436.htm

By changing the way you react to the stressors in your life, you will reprogram your mind & your body. Soon lowering stress levels during your average day will become automatic.

Successful stress management is the key to lowering physical tension in your body.

Notice how you feel when you are exhausted. There is an opposite way to feel—energetic, strong & capable. That is what you are aiming for the majority of the time.

Your goal is to reduce stress on your four pillars of optimal health & fitness: lifestyle, exercise, nutrition & supplementation… & increase their strength.

Think of these as a chain. A chain is only as strong as it's weakest link. If one of the links breaks, the whole chain breaks & the entire system cease's to work.

Stress holds you back from achieving everything you want out of life. I guarantee *that stress management is a skill you want to master.*

Unfortunately, there will be times when *real* stress is evident. For me, this was when my mother was diagnosed first with cancer & then a brain tumor. These moments in my life gave me a whole new perspective on stress.

You must try to alleviate stress any way you can. Sometimes it may not be easy, but it's essential that you attempt to deal with your personal stress, just as I had to deal with mine.

I will provide some useful techniques that you can sprinkle through your week & benefit from for life.

Principle Exercise 3
Thirty-Second Intense Smile

- *Illness-related stress & many other kinds of stress can be managed.*

Sometimes the stress, if not dealt with quickly, can evolve into anger & depression. You must not let this happen.

Instead, at times of repeated stress-triggers you must break the onslaught.

Apply principle 4 - a simple thirty-second smile.

- **Smile & hold it for thirty seconds.** *Take a few deep breaths into this massive smile.*

Smile with your whole face—your eyebrows, cheeks, temple, scalp, eyes, ears, mouth & even tongue. Try it now.

- *Your entire face will find a new position when you focus on smiling intensely. You'll feel better almost instantly. Apply this technique liberally.*
You may look strange to others if you do it in public, but I guarantee you'll feel much better for it.

- *The in-public trick… Lean forward, cup your entire face*
with your hands & smile behind your hands. To onlookers,
you'll look as though you're yawning.

This way, you can complete the exercise many times through your day, no matter where you are.

Principle 3:
I Consistently Uplift My Internal Vibe

Stimulate good vibes from within yourself rather than waiting for external sources to influence you one way or the other.

Imagine for a moment that your happiness is solely dependent on your own internal state & that you have full control over it.

This may seem like a novel thought, but you can make it work for you.

When you stimulate these positive vibes regularly, a new energy will begin to pervade your every experience.

Apply this technique liberally, especially when you are stressed, sad, or even depressed.

Just do it, again & again.

Eventually your vibe will increase & you will be better off for it.

Not only can this make you feel better in the short term, it will also stimulate creativity & a more outgoing personality for the long term.

Trust it. Stick with it… Reap the rewards.

Fake it till you make it.

Get a Handle on Stress

Stress is like a pressure valve. If you don't release it regularly, the pressure will blow—mentally, physically or emotionally.

Even if you perform better under pressure, you still need to deal with the stress so it doesn't negatively impact your body, mind & eventually your spirit.

If you are exhausted, overwhelmed, or physically tense, this is what you can do.

- *De-stress in bed.* What do you usually do there? Make it a sacred, restful pleasure zone, whether you're meditating, sleeping, making love, or just daydreaming (ideally not at the same time!). Work & stress are not permitted here.

- *No phones, no laptops, no devices.* Once in bed, slow down your thoughts. Try to keep your thoughts under control & take long, deep slow breaths. There are only three things you should do in bed: 1) Sleep. 2). Read. 3) Enjoy sex. Everything else should be left for outside of your sacred space, the daytime, not bedtime.

- *Meditate! Even though it may sound "airy fairy" to you, meditation has its benefits.* You can call it whatever you like—try *contemplation*. Slow down your thoughts & your breathing. I suffered for years with migraines & painful, blinding headaches. Meditation (contemplation) stopped the migraines & protected me from further attacks. These daylong attacks no longer stunt my productivity. More about this later.

- *Absorb specific related information. I recommend reading* **How to Achieve Total Success** *by Russ Von Hoelscher &* **The Silva Mind Control Method** *by José Silva.* Both books helped me completely heal myself of the torturous headaches that occurred with increased regularity. Choose a time to meditate that suits you. I do it for a minimum of fifteen minutes daily. Two twenty-minute sessions have been shown to dramatically increase productivity in highly successful people.

- *Make sure you meditate every day.* I found that when I stopped, my headaches returned full force. Your brain needs a break as well & it will let you know when it isn't getting it.

Through daily meditation, I became more positive, more focused & better at breathing, communicating & being mindful—plus I gained more control of runaway cortisol (stress) levels.

I feel great when I take this small amount of time for myself every day. There is a real reason why monks in Asia & successful people the world over focus on meditation. It is a way to connect with yourself & your actual needs.

It will provide you with added vigor, focus & drive.

Principle Exercise 4
Thought Mastery

Read this a few times. Take it in, try it out & repeat it until you know it by heart. Focus on time, posture & your talk-in statement.

- *Go to a room where you will not be disturbed. Make sure nothing will interrupt you.*

- *Sit down, with your back upright. This can be on a chair, on your bed, on the floor or even on the toilet! Place your hands on your knees & relax.*

- *Close your eyes. Do not break your routine.*

- *You are going to develop the ability to visualize in detail & will practice full breathing.*

Small Steps

1. Set your alarm to your chosen time range, such as fifteen to twenty minutes. This must be uninterrupted.

2. Sit, begin to relax & close your eyes.

3. Set a "talk-in" statement—something you say in your head or out loud.

Example

"I am going to meditate, contemplate or simply relax (choose whatever label you prefer), clearing all thoughts from my mind. I am practicing slowing down, having fewer thoughts & being calm. I connect with my energy levels, relax & am recharging with every breath I take."

Once you practice this three to five times, you will have it memorised. As long as what you say is positive & clear, you can't go wrong.

4. Picture an open doorway. See yourself standing in a bright kitchen, with the basement door open. Imagine a spiral staircase leading down to the basement.

5. Slowly start to count down from three to one. While you count & breathe, visualise yourself walking down the staircase.

6. After each number, say, "Counting further; going deeper."

7. Slowly count from three to one. Slow your breathing. When you reach one, imagine arriving on the basement floor & being in the dark room, everything is silent & still.

8. Take one slow deep, breath. Say, "Basic meditation level." Do nothing but focus on the previous statement.

9. Next, say, "Counting further; going deeper" while taking a slow, deep breath.

10. Now count slowly from five to one while breathing slowly & consistently.

11. As you count from five to one, imagine the basement surroundings fading away. As you reach the number one, imagine arriving on a beautiful beach. As you reach one, say, "Reaching a deep meditational state."

12. Take a deep, slow breath. Your eyes are still closed & you are sitting upright, but you are relaxed throughout your body.

13. Take at least twenty slow, deep breaths. As you breathe in, focus on the number one. As you breathe out focus on the number two & so on. If your mind wanders, simply return to your breathing & the last number you remember. Don't get stressed if you start thinking about something else. Just return to the technique.

14. Keep coming back to the number you think you're at. Focus on your breath. Notice it. Deepen each breath. You will eventually master this process & be able to totally relax. It may not be easy to achieve, but it is possible with practice—& totally worth it.

15. Here you have many options. You can choose to just quiet your mind, slow your thoughts & practice being still.

With a little more practice, you can start to intensely focus on areas of your life. For example, you might picture the perfect outcome of an upcoming event. Or you can focus intensely on something you want a solution to. With practice, you can achieve a lot while doing "nothing."

16. Spend as much time as you wish here—from twenty breaths to fifty, or even one hundred breaths. Choose a number & stick to it until you master being able to focus for that period of time. Build up from twenty. Time may be your limiting factor, which is fine. Just master your mind for your set time period using the technique above.

17. It is critical that you keep your eyes shut. Try to keep every part of your body still for the total time you have set. Ignore itches & breathe into any discomfort you may feel. It will not last forever.

18. When you have completed your breaths, or your alarm goes off, slowly bring yourself out of this state.

Practice staying calm, even on the way out. Don't just snap out of it. Slowly bring yourself out using the following sequence to strengthen your "contemplative state," which increases the return on your time investment in this technique.

19. From your deep meditation (contemplation or relaxing) beach, it is time to count out. Picture two steps on the beach. Say, "I am counting out & feeling much better than before."

20. Slowly start to count from one to five. Imagine taking the two steps & beginning to rise off the beach. Float upward, back toward your basement.

21. As you reach the number five, imagine arriving back in your basement.

22. When you reach the basement, say, "Basic meditation state." Take a deep breath in & hold it for a moment & then exhale.

23. Say, "Counting out further. Feeling much better than before. Maintaining connection with my deep meditational state." Now count from one to three, traveling back up the spiral staircase as you do this.

24. When you reach three, step into the brightly lit room & open your eyes. Smile. Say, "I am wide awake, feeling much better than before." Smile.

Principle 4:
I Am The Master Of My Thoughts

Develop your own style of "Contemplation time" (meditation).

Apply this technique daily to gain more control of your mind space - physical, mental & emotional responses to your daily experiences.

After a few attempts, you will start to create your own pattern & further strengthen the control you have over your mind.

With regular practice you can master your mind.

Another benefit of doing this is that you gain greater control over your stress levels. As you read on you will understand how this is critical in this day & age if longevity of your life & success is one of your goals.

You also increase your ability to focus. This has a profound affect over the quality of your work, your conversations & rate of progression in every area of your life.

*Not bad for practicing something so simple.
Make this a religious practice – Never Miss A Day.*

Restore Balance with Tai Chi & Qigong

Slow movements that look like a graceful martial art—this is what characterises Tai Chi & Qigong. You probably know them from seeing groups of people moving together in unison in public parks or studios.

These movements connect your breath & internal focus to rejuvenate the mind & body. This has been proven to lower cholesterol levels, blood pressure & obesity.

According to a study conducted by the *Journal of Alternative and Complementary Medicine*,[3] Tai Chi is health promoting in dozens of ways.

In this study 76 healthy subjects with blood pressure at high normal or stage 1 hypertension underwent a 12-week Tai Chi Chuan exercise-training program.

After this time period the group showed significant decrease in systolic blood pressure & diastolic blood pressure. Cholesterol decreased & high-density lipoprotein (HDL) cholesterol increased (a good thing). Anxiety was also decreased.

These exercises involve slow, rhythmical movements, which encourages blood flow around the body. Blood flow gets more oxygen to your organs & tissues, therefore making you feel more alive & energised.

A single session of Tai Chi or Qigong includes deep breathing for twenty to forty minutes. It has a profound impact on your health!

---

3 Jen-Chen Tsai, Wei-Hsin Wang, Paul Chan, Li-Jung Lin, Chia-Huei Wang, Brian Tomlinson, Ming-Hsiung Hsieh, Hung-Yu Yang, and Ju-Chi Liu. The Journal of Alternative and Complementary Medicine. October 2003, 9(5): 747-754. doi:10.1089/107555303322524599.

In Western society, we are not used to the benefits of deep breathing, but it is so important to good health.

Release the Radicals...

Proper blood circulation is an important part of health. Blood feeds your body with oxygen & nutrients, which promotes natural regeneration of your cells, which improves organ health & function.

Free radicals are atoms or molecules with a single or unpaired electron in the outer shell. This means that it holds the potential to create disharmony within your system.

Free radical damage occurs when the free radical seeks to pair its unpaired electron with another electron. The extra electron is often pulled off of a neighbouring molecule therefore destabilising that electron & in turn making it a free radical.

This can cause a chain of events where the system ends up becoming dysfunctional – a chain reaction of free radical production.

Through its calming & regenerative affect in many ways, Tai Chi is a natural, preventive measure against the damage free radicals in your diet & environment can have on you. Not to mention an ally in the war against stress & fat!

Remember one principle does not cure all. It is the combination of principles within this book that place you in direct alignment with Optimalism.

A healthy diet with ideal amounts of antioxidants will work wonders in combination with regular practice of Tai Chi, meditation or structured relaxation time. Rotate the tools that you use, or find a regular practice of the one, which you feel, of most benefit to you.

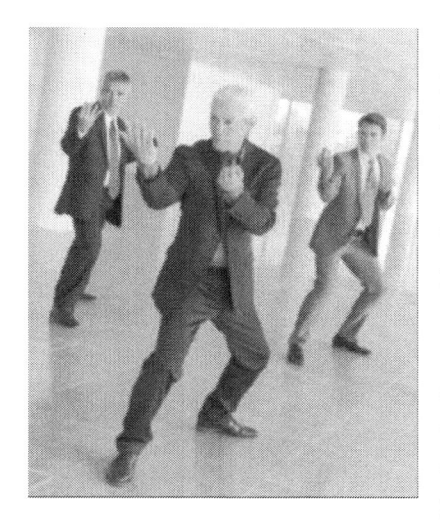

Tai Chi & Qigong are internal martial arts that promote a healthier mind-body connection.

Find yourself a Tai Chi or Qigong teacher, join a class, buy a DVD, or invest in a book.

There are many books & DVDs available to get you started. Tai Chi & Qigong are easier than other forms of exercise in that they are more of an internal exercise.

We could label them working in. Whereas a weight training, or sprint training session is definitely exerting energy outwards.

Tai Chi is the practice of pulling energy or promoting the growth of energy from within.

Either way these forms of exercise certainly have their place within a balanced lifestyle.

Trust me when I say that you should not miss out on the benefits that they have to offer.

If stress is a disease, then Tai Chi, Qigong & meditation are vaccines.

Make a Difference

Do something out of routine. This can have a positive impact on your stress levels.

- Change your routine. Simple things like getting out of bed on the opposite side you usually do, brush your teeth with the opposite hand, or shower using a scrubbing brush rather than a sponge or your bare hands.

- *Alter your usual routes to work, your children's schools & your favourite restaurants.*

- Changing your routine makes you happier. When you do something different or new, dopamine production is stimulated. Dopamine is a hormone & neurotransmitter that is related to mood & focus. Break your daily cycles & try new things to increase your production of dopamine.

- Write about your experience; it is incredibly therapeutic. Sorting out what is in your subconscious by bringing it into the physical world by writing it down helps you make sense of things, which is a huge de-stressor. This is effectively what you do when you dream – you process what is swimming round your subconscious. Give yourself a head start by getting the traffic jam out of your head. This will help you get an even better night's sleep.

- Be aware of the language you use to talk to yourself. You wouldn't allow anyone else to be disrespectful to you so do not do it to yourself. As a successful person you are likely very critical of yourself, I'd bet that sometimes you can be over critical. Make your subconscious mind a fortress by guiding your conscious mind toward positivity or worst-case scenario use constructive criticism on yourself.

- Communicate with other people & make new friends. Get out & see the world through the eyes of new people. The quickest way to have a new experience is to meet a group of people who are doing something different.

- Positive conversation with anyone is an absolute de-stressor. Sometimes a simple action can help a situation.

"A problem shared is a problem halved."

When you feel burdened & stressed, talk about it. Get those feelings out of your head & body. Talk into your phone, talk out loud in your car or a private place, talk to a friend, family member, colleague etc., whoever you feel you can vent to – the trick is to allow your stress out without any resistance.

Talk into an empty space or to a good listener. You'd be amazed at what a full out shout or scream can do for your stress levels… however maybe don't try this in the middle of the office!

Chapter 4:
Renew Yourself
Once & For All

Renewal requires opening yourself up to new ways of thinking and feeling.

—Deborah Day
Author, mental health clinician

Stress, fatigue & living an unhealthy lifestyle can be taxing beyond anything we could imagine. Now we understand the far-reaching effects of our behavior, thanks to scientific & medical research.

This chapter focuses on renewal—mentally, physically & emotionally. At this stage, you'll make new decisions that will affect who you are.

This is not a good thing—it's a great thing. Even more positive experiences are within your reach.

Review Your View

As the final part *of the first step* in the LENS Wellness System, consider your life as it is right now. You already know how important review & analysis can be in the future success of a department or company.

Reviewing your life does the same thing. It allows you to seize & replicate the successes & eliminate the mistakes. One size does not fit all. If it did, there would only be one diet book in the world & no need for any other.

- Review what eating plans have worked for you & what ones have not. Make a clear note of what plan worked for you in the past – if any?

- Are your food choices driven by taste or nutrition? You will be changing to food choices that are driven by how they make your body function & feel, rather than just about how the food tastes.

- Know yourself well. Take responsibility for how you have behaved in the past. The real trick will be to understand why you behave the way you do, whether you deem each behavior positive or negative, it is still helpful to understand why you chose to behave in the way you do. Whether it's a weekly, monthly, or annual review, track your decisions & behaviors over big decisions in your life. You can start to do this today by making notes in your phone, on your laptop, or in a note pad.

- *Achieving your goals relies on your ability to understand yourself & your reactions to each situation.* When you do, you can anticipate mistakes, pitfalls & failures—& then actively avoid them leading to even greater success.

  Everyone needs a coach. Professional athletes have coaches & so do professional singers, chefs & top business people. It's important to be accountable to someone for your actions. Search for a coach for area(s) of your life where you know you can be better.

Be honest with yourself, if you are not already. This approach will serve you well in the long run. I have no hesitation in seeking out someone who knows more than me about a subject & picking their brains, or paying them for their time. Learn more to earn more – this is an old saying that always runs true. Learn the lessons that can scale you upwards & onwards ASAP & live a happier life.

Principle Exercise 5
ShapeTrainer Review Wheel

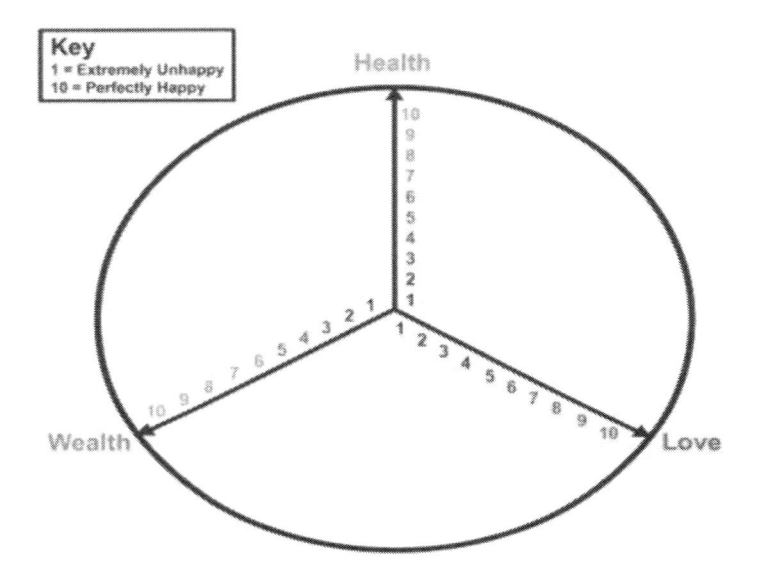

Health, Wealth & Love – Once a person is satisfied with these three areas of their life they will be at peace.

- *Rate yourself from one to ten using the review wheel above.One = unhappy/dissatisfied*

Ten = happy/completely satisfied.

Once you rate each area, join your selected numbers with a line, following the shape of the outer circle as you draw the line.

You will create an internal circle related to your personal scores for each section.

- *The shape your numbers create highlights the balance in your life. In an ideal world. You will have created a perfect wheel—you circled ten for each area. This makes a wheel that, when placed on the road, flows smoothly along its path.*

If your results resemble a triangle, you will have a bumpy ride.

- *This exercise highlights the area, or areas, that you need to focus on most. Once you improve your scores, your life will flow more smoothly.*

- *The goal is to make this wheel perfectly round so that things run smoothly. Also, the larger your wheel, the better.*

You will cover more ground with greater ease.

Note: Once you achieve the highest possible scores for each area of your review wheel, you'll notice it resembles a peace symbol.

Once you have organised your life to achieve top scores in these areas, your daily life experience will also appear more peaceful.

This exercise is to point out areas of focus. As the premise of this book is health & fitness you would think that the principles within would only help the health section of the review wheel.

What you will find is that as you improve your health, your ability to learn, earn, love & all the other facets of being human will also be heightened. It cannot fail to have effect.

Improve one are of your life & you positively affect every other area at the same time.

Principle 5:
I Live At The Peak Of Health, Wealth & Love

Apply the exercises & techniques in this book to slowly, but surely, increase your review wheel scores.

If you manage to apply all of the principles that you have been supplied with so far, you will immediately notice a shift beginning to happen in your day-to-day life. Maybe others will notice something different about you?

The more you apply the principles the more you can benefit from their inherent power.
Some are extremely subtle but they have far reaching effects across your life.

Once you complete this book, or in a few weeks' time, retest your personal score across the review wheel

If you have a low score in one area, focus on that area for a period of time. Again, use the exercises & principles provided herein to continually improve your scores (status).

Do what is necessary to bring each score up.
The other areas of your life will benefit as a result.

Renew Your Energy Levels Quickly

Let's get serious again. Some days your energy may be bottoming out, you feel like someone pours you out of bed & into your clothes & the rest is autopilot.

I know that feeling.

There are six core methods for instantly improving your dwindling energy levels that you can integrate into every day.

1. **Keep Your Thoughts Positive.**
   When you think & speak in a positive manner, you create positive experiences around you. Instant energy. No matter how you feel make sure that the language you use is always on the positive side.

2. **Practice Proper Breathing.**
   Breathe deeply & rhythmically to become calm. The calmer you are, the less stress you feel. Adequate oxygen in your blood & brain does a lot to ease muscle stress & improve performance so that you can achieve maximum productivity & output.

3. **Hydrate.**
   Even 1 percent dehydration can cause a significant drop in performance levels. Drink at least 1.5 liters (approx. 6 cups) of clean, filtered water every twenty-four hours. If you weigh more than 50 kg, (110lbs) you will need more for optimal results. If you exercise intensely, you will require even more. Even in cool laboratory conditions, maximal aerobic power (VO2max) decreases by about 5% when persons experience fluid losses equivalent to 3% of body mass or more (Pinchan et al. 1988).

4. Be Nicely Nourished.
Correct your diet & give your body the nutrients it needs to thrive. Eat a good breakfast & then eat consistently throughout the day to keep your body fuelled with the right amount of nutrients. Without nutrients, your body runs on empty. We'll talk more about this later.

5. Sleep Like a Log.
You should feel rested & energised when you wake up. If you don't, the quality of your sleep is not optimal & this will in turn have affect over your day. For improved performance in the morning, get more sleep before midnight. The truth is that less than six hours is simply too little sleep. More about this later.

6. *Nurture a Rich Internal Life*
Spend time alone so that you can contemplate & review your day in peace. You must integrate 'quiet time' into your day – as explained above, refer to Principle 5 as an example of this. A jam-packed day with no time alone is not a healthy day. You will be fine for a while, maybe even some years but eventually this will catch up with you – but it doesn't have to.

Even ten minutes of meditation (contemplation) can help refocus your mind on productivity. I highly recommend taking at least thirty minutes of alone time for reflection each day.

Eliminate Subconscious Hurdles

Along with the above methods, you can also review your internal thoughts about money.

Eliminate the little things that keep bugging you, like creating a will. That can add stress to your life without you even realising where it's coming from.

After years of dealing with successful individuals, I've found that getting info out of your head is the key. Get the constant swirl of to-dos out of your mind by writing them down. Using notes on your phone is a simple & effective method of doing this.

Write everything down that pops into your mind that needs completing. Once you've completed one task, delete it & move on to the next.

You don't have to remember everything. Take a load off wherever possible.

Thought Control for Greater Results

In a chain of movement, the weakest link always breaks when the system is put under an overload of stress.

Physical pain causes kinks—a muscle injury, joint pain, or a torn ligament. Mental overload can also cause imbalances & weaknesses or eventual breakdown.

You have to learn to control your thought patterns to gain maximum control over the physical world & your body.

Life happens whether you prepare for it or not. Do you know anyone who is not affected by stress in one-way or another? Highly unlikely.

There is no way you can avoid stress forever, but you can prepare for it & manage it.

A large part of that preparation & management is attached to your thought patterns – the more positive your language & self talk the less stressed you will feel, no matter what is going on.

- ***Think about what you are thinking.***
  Separate yourself from the cyclical thoughts in your mind. Your brain is trying to understand & process information. You can help it by distancing yourself from your thoughts & consciously segmenting them. Notice that you are in fact not your thoughts. They are a mechanism that functions as part of you, but they are not you in totality.

If you learn to separate your reactionary thoughts to everyday stimulus, you can control your day-to-day life experiences from an internal viewpoint. Thought patterns work to shape & frame how you experience the world, but this can be under your control. It begins by taking ownership & control of a single thought.

- ***Often your thoughts contradict your goals & you don't even realise it.***
  You can use your mind as a tool to improve your life, or make it a misery. I strongly suggest you practice making it a paradise.

Everyone in the world has a connection & reaction to each word. Saying, "Yes," inspires you to be ready, while saying, "No," does the opposite. Notice the feeling within when you say the word no. Say the word out loud or in your head, try it now. Then notice how you feel when you say yes. Feel the difference.

In most cases, when a person says, "No," they will feel a subtle drop in energy & could feel less powerful. Except when that person is being taken advantage of, then the word ***no*** becomes an increase in energy & power. That is how strong words can be. But be very aware of the subtlety of context. The same word can be negative in most situations & position in others!

- ***Thoughts are made up of words & images that we internalise.***
  Learn to tell yourself the truth, to motivate yourself & to stay fiercely positive. Positivity is like a mirror. It comes back to you in reality. Negativity is like a black hole that sucks you in & drains you of vital energy.

If you have not already - you must begin positive thought spirals in your life.

They will boost your energy levels, support your immune system & remove blockages to greater levels of success in every area of your life.

Principle Exercise 6
Positive Alphabet

- *Focus on how you feel at this very moment— energetic/lethargic, happy/sad, focused/distracted & so on.*

- *Make a mental note of your current emotional, physical & mental state.*

- *Get comfortable—sitting, standing, wherever you are.*

Now think of a positive word starting with the letter A— For example, achievement or awesome.

- *Do the same for B, C & D, all the way through the alphabet.*

- *Once you have completed the entire alphabet, review how you feel.*

Is there a difference in your emotional, physical, or mental state from when you began the exercise?

- *Within only a few minutes something as simple as this can uplift you.*

It's easy & anyone can do it.

- *Words are powerful. "Words are things," so be conscious & deliberate in which words you choose to represent you every day. When you talk to others – externally & to yourself – internally.*

- *This includes words you use in your internal dialogue—the words you use to talk to yourself, the ones no one else can hear.*

Notice if you talk to yourself using positive or negative internal dialogue/words.

- *The progression of this exercise is to make your internal dialogue more positive than it currently is.*

Principle 6
I Use Positive Language Always, in All Ways.

There is a root to everything. Thoughts can program behavior. Images, words & language structure thought.

Thoughts are the root of instruction from your brain to your body.

Learn to control them by first learning how to influence them.

By consciously choosing your words, thoughts, & actions you slowly but surely create the experience of your life that you truly desire rather than being at the whim of habit or what you happened to learn growing up.

Do you notice negative patterns of thinking within yourself?

You may notice that you talk to yourself in a negative way sometimes? This can be called internal dialogue.

The healthier, more positive & supportive this dialogue is the happier & healthier you will feel.

This will likely not solve the entire puzzle of your life but it is a massive piece of the puzzle that you must get handled.

Be in control of your words. Consciously choose your language so that is benefits you.

Breathe to Achieve

How often are you aware of the *way* that you breathe?

I you are like most people that is not often. You most likely become consciously aware of your breathing when you run upstairs or are suddenly anxious.

Breathing may be an autonomic process, but the conscious mind can & *must* influence it from time to time.

You breathe according to your personality. If you are a laid-back person, you likely enjoy deep, rhythmical breathing. If you are a nervous, angry, or frustrated person, you are probably prone to shallow, erratic & faster breathing patterns.

When a person suffers a severe injury & emergency services are called, the call center ranks the priority of the call (injury):

1. *Breathing*
2. *Bleeding*
3. *Burns*
4. *Bones*

If your breathing is interrupted for a prolonged period of time, you are in deep trouble. So the emergency services rank breathing related injuries as high priority.

Detached limbs may be successfully reattached after 6 hours of no blood circulation at warm temperatures. Bone, tendon, & skin can survive as long as 8 to 12 hours.[1]

---

1 Replantaion at eMedicine. http://en.wikipedia.org/wiki/EMedicine

The most vulnerable cells in the brain, CA1 neurons of the <u>hippocampus</u>, are fatally injured by as little as 10 minutes without oxygen[2]

This illustrates the importance of optimal breathing. Granted you wont need medical attention if you hold your breath for a few seconds or don't breathe perfectly for a day or so!

However, the fact remains that the closer to optimal your breathing patterns the closer to optimal the function of your brain & body.

This leads to the possibility that if you breathe more effectively most of the time you will likely perform at a higher level – mentally & physically.

You can very easily apply this basic principle to day. Monitor & address your internal climate or situation through breathing.

Any condition caused by stress—tight muscles, lack of energy, laziness, fatigue, abdominal pain, back pain, dizziness etc.— will negatively affect your breathing pattern. Or vice versa - If your breathing is affected, these conditions can appear exaggerated.

The good news is that you can consciously change those patterns that promote an unhealthy mind-set, body, or lifestyle & free yourself from these blockages.

---

2 Kirino T, T (2000). "Delayed neuronal death". *Neuropathology* **20**: S95–7. doi:10.1046/j.1440-1789.2000.00306.x. PMID 11037198.

Principle Exercise 7
Conscious Deep Diaphragmatic Breath

• *Lie down on your back & get comfortable. Place your hands just below your ribs. Focus on your hands while you take deep breathes. The goal is to make your hands rise as high as possible when you breathe in.*

• *Become breath-aware. Be conscious of the way you breathe & try to make each breath full & deep. Practice this pattern every day. After a couple of times lying down, try it sitting up & then standing.*

• *Expand your rib cage as much as possible with every inhalation.*

• *For every exhalation, push all the air from your lungs.*

• *Exaggerate every breath to its maximum—in & out.*

• *Complete ten to one hundred breaths with this technique, remaining focused throughout.*

• *You may fall asleep, so it may be helpful to set an alarm. If you do fall asleep, that's OK. You have successfully relaxed yourself & this is a good thing.*

Some Added Extras:

• *Practice nose breathing—in through your nose & out through your nose. Breathing in & out through your nose makes you take a deeper breath. It automatically encourages you to fill your lungs with each breath.*

• Practice breathing in through your nose & out through your mouth. Try to keep it at four seconds for each inhalation & four for each exhalation. Try this technique the next time you're tired, nauseous, or ill. It can help because it increases oxygen in your blood, it will make you feel grounded & calm.

• Practice holding your breath for a few seconds. On each breath, inhale & hold for three to ten seconds. Then exhale & hold no breath for three to ten seconds. Repeat five to ten times.

*• **Exaggerate your breathing.** Breathe deeply through your nose & out hard through your mouth - ten to twenty times in a row.*

• Practice exaggerated breathing above & prolonging the exhaled position. This useful breath-control exercise helps strengthen your breathing pattern. After approximately 2 minutes of this return to normal breathing, make a mental note of how this makes you feel.

Principle 7:
I Breathe Optimally

*To improve your performance & essentially your health,
there are few things better for you than optimal breathing patterns.*

*Improving breath patterns will improve your performance at work,
home & every other area of your life.*

*Deep breathing can help relax you at any point in the day
or before bed to help you have a good night's sleep.*

*Master conscious breathing so you become fully aware of when you
are not breathing for optimal health & performance.*

*After injecting some conscious practice into your day, optimal
breathing will become automatic once again.*

*Like a sleeping baby your lungs should fill with air, your ribcage rise
with each inhalation, relaxing further with every breath.*

*With each exhalation you de-stress, flowing tension along with
toxins out & away from your body.*

Your mind is sharpened through consistent optimal breathing.

*You place yourself in line with success & the process is fully
within your control.*

*When you breathe optimally you reduce your stress levels & free
you mind to focus more intensely. These two benefits go a long way
to propelling you toward optimal health & fitness.*

Sleep Is Medicine

Sleep is the body's way of shutting down for a period of repair, mentally reviewing & processing experiences from your day & preparing for the next day, or moments ahead.

You only stand a chance of being at your absolute best when you achieve optimal sleep patterns. Only then are you primed to achieve physical & mental perfection—or get as close to it as possible.

- *You spend a third of your life sleeping.*
  Sleep must be important if this much of your life is taken up by it. In my opinion, quality sleep is the most overlooked variable in health, fitness & physical performance levels. Sleep affects your body in hundreds of ways that science is still trying to fully understand.

- *Sleep improves your response to exercise.*
  Sleep can become your own "anabolic steroid response" to training. You will boost growth hormone, lower cortisol & recover fully from stress & exercise when you get quality sleep. Growth hormone is a hormone that stimulates growth, cell reproduction & regeneration. It can be affected by your sleep patterns.

- *Poor quality sleep inhibits your body's healing response.*
  To properly heal from infection, viruses, bacteria, injury & other external forces, you must get adequate sleep. Inadequate sleep will lower your immune system. If your immune system is impaired you will be physically weaker. If you are physically weaker you will not be able to work as hard in the gym & will not achieve your full potential of progression.

- *Sleep is a crucial piece of the healthy lifestyle puzzle.*
  Ignore it at your own peril. Or, even better, try getting high quality sleep for one solid week. Write down how you feel. You will never go back to scrimping on the number of hours & quality of your sleep. The positive effects will be far reaching.

- *Sleep deprivation is a common modern disorder.*
  So is not following set sleeping rituals & patterns. Your body yearns for a good sleep routine. Set this up & you'll set yourself up for greater success. Your body will find optimum quickly once you begin to follow a regular circadian rhythm. This is the rhythm of your sleep – wake cycles. The more regular & stable they are the more optimally your body & brain will function.

The old saying, *"Early to bed, early to rise makes a man healthy, wealthy & wise"* will always ring true. This is because it is a principle of health that you experience regular quality sleep.

Why do you think sleep deprivation has been used as a torture over the years! If your sleeping patterns are poor it is time to stop torturing yourself.

Make sure that you get enough sleep—numerous studies show that at least seven to nine hours each evening, *every evening are the ideal amount for optimal brain & body activity.*

Add optimal sleep patterns, naps & routines to your daily regimen how you see fit or how you know work best for you.

Install a calming routine before bed & then drift off at around the same time each night to wake at around the same time each morning.

Aligning your sleep with nature (natural light & melatonin production) is best.

Melatonin is a hormone associated with deep sleep & circadian rhythms. It is a powerful antioxidant & protects your mitochondrial DNA (converting energy from food into a form that cells can use).

Circadian rhythm is the natural cycle of the sun & moon. When it gets dark, you relax & go to sleep. As it gets light, you wake & progress through your day.

If you get broken sleep every night, it's important to isolate the reason why & resolve it. When you don't sleep straight through the night, your body cannot effectively repair itself. That means any physical or psychological recovery is impaired for the next day.

Your production of melatonin is disrupted by only three seconds of being awake. If this happens on a regular basis, you are missing out on the rewards that deep sleep has to offer. Prolonged absence of the deep sleep that melatonin offers can be a cause of immune suppression & eating disorders [1]

So if you regularly get ill or have trouble sticking to a healthy eating plan, try getting to sleep earlier, you'll be amazed at how well this helps strengthen your will power.

Use the "ShapeTrainer SSSSH Principles" to improve your sleep:

Shut out electricity,
Seal off noise,
Stop all stimulants,
Supplement Your Sleep
Harness the Power of the Dark.

---

1 http://www.sleepeducation.com/news/2012/07/05/sleep-loss-triggers-stress-like-immune-response

1) Shut out all electricity.

An ultraviolet light the size of a pin tip shone on the sole of your foot will bring you out of a deep sleep!

What does this mean? It means that the quality of your sleep can easily be reduced. You must protect yourself from this. Sleep is prompted by natural cycles of activity in the brain & consists of two basic states: rapid eye movement (REM) sleep & non-rapid eye movement (NREM) sleep, which consists of 4 stages.

Stages 1 to 4 are increasing depth of sleep state. If you progress through all 4 stages smoothly & spend optimal time within each phase the better you will repair & recover.

The better you sleep, the more productive you will be & the more you align yourself with success. A little effort spent improving your sleep patterns is worth it.

Think about all the electrical equipment you have in your bedroom. That's not to mention all the Wi-Fi options that are buzzing through you. We'll address those in a moment.

Helpful

The more electrical interference there is, the more stress there will be on your body & mind. If you feel overrun, or have ever felt this way, then reducing this stress is extremely helpful.

How do you do that? First, be aware of all the electrical equipment in your bedroom. Second, unplug everything in your room. Only plug it in when you want to use it.

This will put a stop to any LCD light displays interrupting the depth of your sleep & any electrical interference that equipment could be chucking off.

Again, I stress that you must reap the benefits of sleep by using your sleep patterns like medicine.

A Small Solution

In this day & age, we are surrounded—bombarded, even—by electrical impulses in our environment. There's no escaping it. So a sensible approach would be to manage your exposure or your response to certain exposure.

Why not take any & every step to improve your health & performance levels?

Even if the method of protection has a minimal effect on your health, it will gather momentum & be well worth it in the long run. When you combine a number of small positive & effective techniques, you get an accumulation of benefits.

"The whole is greater than the sum of the parts"

—Kurt Koffka.

This sentence explains the importance of Optimalsm as a whole. You may look at one of the principles of Optimalism & wonder what benefits it may bring to your life?

However in combination the 24 principles of Optmalism are profound. Once you autonomise them within your life they will begin to work as a symphony. Each principle performing at the perfect time to create a master piece which is your life.

Each principle bringing you back to balance & consistently on the road to greater success in body & mind.

Save Yourself…

Imagine filling your car with fuel. You drive around from A to B & clearly see your fuel gauge going down. Imagine fitting something to your car that makes it more fuel-efficient.

In the first day of doing this, you save a small amount of fuel. After one month, however, you may have saved a whole tank.

Spread that over years, even decades & you get an idea of how you can save energy, health & vitality by applying small techniques, methods & devices to your life.

Remember that when you apply a number of seemingly small, pointless things to your life, they have an accumulative effect.

If the things are negative—such as eating food wrapped in plastic & slowly absorbing small amounts of that into your body—then the end result will more likely be disease or ill health.

But if the things are positive, de-stressing & protective, then the end result will more likely be optimal health, vitality & freedom.

The same subtle principle applies to the quality of your sleep.

Time to Stop

Stop working on your laptop & phone *at least* two hours before going to bed. In fact, turn off all electrical equipment, including the lights. Does that mean you should stumble around in the dark in order to be healthy? No, but reduce stimulation in the evenings, particularly when you are asleep.

At least turn the lights down to dim, if you can, or replace them with candles. This type of light is more natural & less of a stress on your body. You will also find it more relaxing for your mind.

Most people find it impossible to not watch TV or be on their laptop right up until they decide it's time to go to sleep. They switch everything off & lie in bed, wondering why they can't get to sleep. Maybe you are like this.

Just as a sportsperson prepares themself for the big game, you must prepare for "the big sleep" (optimal sleep).

A useful way to improve your sleeping pattern is to manage your cortisol throughout the day.

Remember cortisol is your stress hormone & should not be stimulated 24/7.

Here's an example of a good cortisol curve. Your cortisol (stress hormone) should fluctuate in a similar pattern in order for you to be at your best, sleep well & perform well.

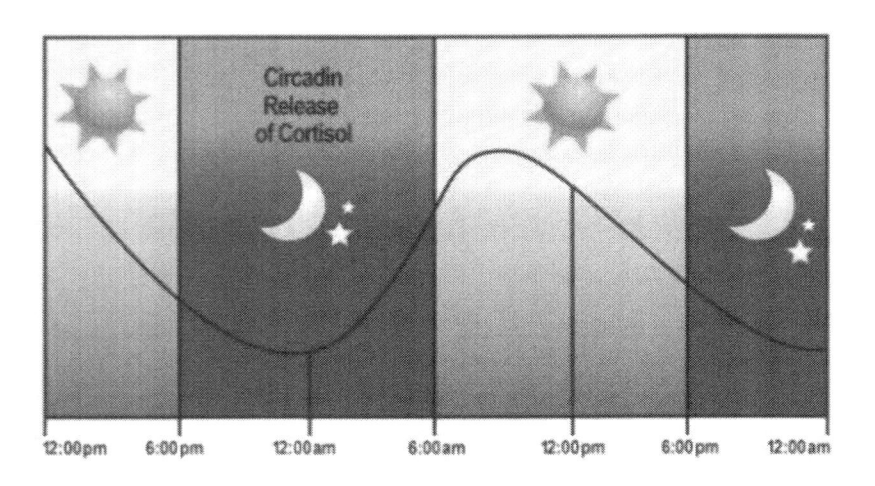

Support your sleep with your decisions around bedtime & throughout your day. Ideally, this means you begin to wind-down from high stress at around 6pm & cease all work by eight thirty at the latest.

This way, you align yourself with greater success. Ideally you are asleep by the ideal golden time of ten thirty.

Obviously, the longer you can give yourself to wind down before you attempt to go to sleep, the better. If you follow the flow of ideal cortisol, your workday should look something like the above diagram. Busy times between 6am & 6pm.

What To Do...

So if you are in a dimly lit room with no TV & no laptop, what do you do? The answer is relax. Be there, not needing to be stimulated by something for a small portion of your day. I'm talking about a few minutes here.

You can mentally run through your day. You can converse with your partner or whomever you live with. You can literally just stretch—think of how a cat simply relaxes & stretches. That's right"—stretch out the stresses of your day. Read, or do whatever you consider relaxing—just be honest with yourself.

What is missing for most people these days is the ability to just be—to be able to sit & do nothing. Nothing required. You should already be practicing this from earlier principles.

When you say it out loud, it sounds stupid, but if you pay attention to most people, you'll notice it's true. They need constant stimulation or they will be bored or unhappy.

How natural is it for babies to just sit & play with nothing more than their own feet or whatever is in sight? They can have fun out of nothing. You can too.

At some point, most people lost the ability to have fun from nothing, to be satisfied with just sitting & doing nothing for one or two hours of their days.

This is what we are missing & what you need to apply to your life in order to relax, de-stress & (very importantly) sleep well.

2) Seal off all noise

When you sleep, your environment should be totally silent. Imagine that you're a caveman. You are in your cave by nine o'clock at the latest & it's dark. Maybe you discovered fire, so you have a few logs burning, but that is relaxing & warm.

Other than the crack of wood burning on your open fire, noise levels are low & there is stillness & moments of silence. It's dark. As your fire slowly burns out, all noise disappears. You are now lying in your cave in the pitch black & in relative silence. Your body relaxes & you go to sleep.

Your cave creates a hollow surrounding that is insular & safe. Your sleep is deep & undisturbed. There are no sounds of buses passing by outside or drunk teenagers arguing, or even the fuzzy sound of a busy road in the distance. It is quiet.

This is the scenario you must replicate for your sleep conditions. I'm not saying you have to sell your house & move into a cave.

A very simple solution is earplugs. They are the easiest & most effective way to seal your ears off to the world for a few minutes or even hours. You'll instantly notice that you sleep better & feel more rested when you wake up.

When was the last time you experienced total silence?

Difference

The difference in how rested I feel when I wear earplugs is remarkable. A deep healing that can happen in the silence.

If you have been skiing or snowboarding you may have noticed the silence on the lift or as you get higher up the mountain. You may have noticed at the top of the lift how still & quiet it is. If you take a moment to realise how your body feels, you'll notice a deep calm.

This deep calm, if allowed, will increase your energy levels from the inside out. When you sit to rest for a moment in the silence, close your eyes & feel the effect it has on your body & mind.

Now bring that experience into your space whenever you want. Earplugs are direct access to that surrounding silence. Think about your day from the moment you wake up. There is noise pollution everywhere around you, especially if you live in the center of a big city like London or New York.

In order to give yourself the best chance of achieving your full potential, you must integrate complete silence into your day—every day.

You can do this through the earlier mind-control techniques to ensure it happens when you go to sleep each night.

If you combine these techniques with earplugs, you'll notice a stillness building within you. From that stillness, you will make better decisions about your health, diet, relationships, jobs, hobbies & every area of your life.

Even the smallest sound can wake some people, while others say that nothing wakes them. If you are one of the latter, consider that the depth of your sleep can be interrupted without you consciously being aware of it.

If this happens on a regular basis, then your sleep is compromised; therefore, so are the results in your life.

Your health, effectiveness, productivity & level of success will be affected sooner, rather than later. Why not deal with this before it becomes an issue? It's a simple adjustment.

The better you sleep, the better you perform when you're awake.

3) Stop all stimulants

Any stimulant you take has a life span. The longer the life span of the stimulant, the longer before you can fully relax. Stimulants can be beneficial, as long as you use them at the right time.

Let's take caffeine as an example, as it is so popular. It takes approximately six hours for the effects of caffeine to fully leave your system.

The initial kick starts to subside after about ten to fifteen minutes for most people. However the effects still course through your veins even when you stop being consciously aware of them.

Your adrenal glands are stimulated for up to six hours from one espresso shot of caffeine. This means that it is impossible for your body to go into full repair & relaxation mode for six hours. This is a massive problem, as coffee is not the only stimulant in play for many people.

Most important is *when* you consume coffee. Late night coffee after dinner can be damaging to your health. Particularly from its affect of keeping you awake or not fully allowing your body to relax & experience optimal sleep, which as you know affects your immune system.

Relax, Unwind, Rest

The main issue is that most people—& this may include you right now—are not able to relax, unwind & rest properly. This causes your body to accumulate stress over time.

When your body is under an accumulation of stress, it eventually starts to malfunction. You may experience an inability to sleep, illness, a physical injury, mental agitation, or unhappiness for no particular reason.

If you have been unhappy & are not sure why, this accumulation of stress could be part of the problem. Refer to the stress section for more detail of the effects of stress & how to reduce it.

If you combine a number of stimulants, like sugar, artificial light, computers & working into the early hours of the morning, then you increase your chances of ill health & unhappiness in the long run.

You have a choice to break this pattern & begin an upward spiral of health & wellness

Quality of Sleep

You may think that alcohol is a stimulant, due to its effects on your body. However, it is actually a depressant. This doesn't mean it's OK to consume alcohol before bed. It affects the quality of your sleep & in the long run leads to a similar place as the stimulants.

If you consume something—anything—that stimulates your body or mind before you go to bed, then you are doing yourself an injustice. You are not supporting yourself to be your best. If you are unhappy with any area of your life, address this now.

When you are fully rested—optimally rested—you have the energy & health funds to give your all. You hold onto the fuel that powers you toward your personal best. If you burn this fuel, you will not have the maximum get-up-&-go. It is subtle, but powerful.

It gives you the extra energy within a conversation. Having the energy to communicate with vigor & enthusiasm could be the difference between success & failure. Resting & preparing to rest optimally gives you "get-up-&-go" with no hesitation. It gives you the ability to concentrate intensely for long periods of time. It gives you greater control in difficult situations. It gives you the feeling of more time to respond & the ability to produce quality thought time & time again.

Gateway

Controlling the stimulants that enter your body is one gateway to these benefits. When you combine all the tips & suggestions in this book, you'll experience a dramatic shift in your level of effectiveness.

The great thing about improving your health, step-by-step, is that you will be rewarded. Within the realm of your own health, no good deed goes unrewarded.

Each healthy application you apply has exponential affects to the quality of your entire life.

Keep applying these techniques to each specific area of your life & your level of enjoyment will increase; your luck will improve & your experiences will expand in a positive way.

It's natural for this to happen to a healthy, happy person. You can continue to control & can improve your life. Improve your health & you will improve everything that occurs to you. When you are at optimal health & fitness you will always lift the spirits & mood of everyone you come into contact with.

Stimulants Are Good

There are, however, times when stimulants benefit you. The general rule of thumb is to use certain stimulants early in the day. This way they can do their job, you can reap the benefits & they can leave your system in time for you to get a solid night's sleep.

Follow the flow of night & day as nature intended. In the morning, when the sun rises, you rise. Your cortisol levels also rise from the point you wake up until around midday. This helps you maintain a high level of productivity. This is when you could apply stimulants without adverse effects.

This should be the busiest, most productive portion of your day. After this time, both you & your workload should begin to slow down. From 6pm onwards you want to begin your decent into relaxation & ending up in bed at a reasonable hour.

This is idealistic thinking & not possible for most who live in the fast lane. *But*, I want to give you the ideal so that you know exactly what the ideal is. You can then choose how you structure your life in relation to ideal & optimal results.

Ideal

As soon as you become aware of the ideal applications of the work-rest-play balance, you'll likely make some small changes to your day. These changes have a subtle effect.

Over time, you'll accumulate momentum in a healthy direction & eventually you may end up living a perfectly healthy life.

If not, at least you'll improve your health & possibly your lifespan, as a by-product.

Use stimulants to your advantage early in the day. Don't consume caffeine, sugar, or other stimulant after four thirty.

Eat clean, drink water & give yourself small breaks. The food, beverages, rest & stimulants you had earlier in the day should carry you through to the end of your day.

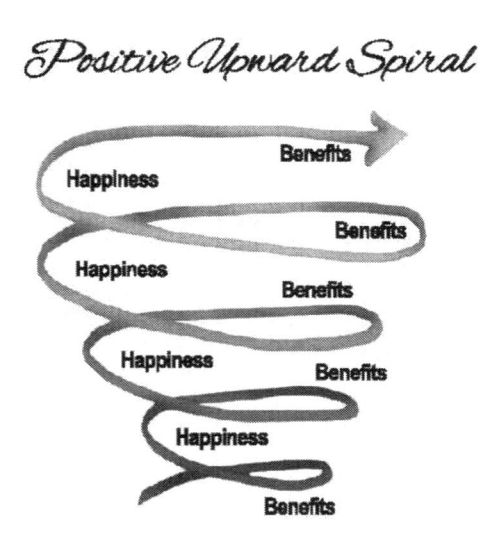

Positive Upward Spiral

We'll go into more detail later in the book about exactly what to eat.

Why four thirty? This gives you six hours to detox & wash out before you go to sleep.

Remember, ten thirty is your ideal sleep cutoff time. If you follow this suggestion, you'll eventually begin to sleep better, followed by better recovery, improved immunity & strength, allowing for improved performance the next day.

Rather than a vicious circle of negative effects that keep dragging you down, you can create a virtuous circle of positive effects that pull you up. Again you have a choice.

Last Point

At this point you may have the thought of immediately ceasing consumption of all stimulants. A word of warning: If you have been using stimulants to get through your day for a long time, it won't be easy to go cold turkey. There's no easy way round it. You'll have to resist your usual overload of caffeine, or your stimulant of choice.

The process of reducing stimulants to help you get through your day will likely get worse before it gets incredibly better.

Instead, do the obvious—cut back slowly. First don't consume any stimulants after four thirty. That's your starting point.

This may mean you're tired later in the day. If so, allow you to be a little tired & take a power nap or small breaks as required to get through. This dip in energy will pass with time as long as you are consistently applying the principles from this book to improve your state of health.

Use principle 5 – Master Your Thoughts. This is a practice of relaxing & focusing. Do this first, before you cave into any craving.

If the craving is unbearable, even after re-applying principle 5 & you just cannot resist, be mindful of what you have & how it makes you feel.

Does it really help & do you feel good for it? How about the next morning? Do you feel that you are getting healthier each day? If you're not, why not?

Good Day

You may bounce around for a while, having one good day & then a bad day. This is natural & normal for most people.

You'll probably know people who can go cold turkey & cut out all stimulants like flicking a switch. They may be less addicted than you are or are already at rock bottom & it just feels right to make the switch in that way.

Again, you must do what is right for you & (most importantly) what works for you.

You may be one of these people mentioned above. If so, go with it.

If not, go with the flow. Do what you need to in order to stay on track toward optimal health & fitness. Release yourself from the stimulant roundabout.

Here are some ideas that help with overcoming stimulant addiction:

   i. Learn how to meditate.
   I have provided you with a foundation technique: Principle 5. Apply this daily, particularly right before you give in to a craving.

   ii. Exercise daily.
   Mark A. Smith, PhD, of Davidson College presented research in San Diego at Neuroscience 2010, the annual meeting for the Society of Neuroscience.
      He showed studies recently completed that individuals who are enrolled in exercise during a formal treatment program are more successful at maintaining abstinence[1]
   More about exercise later in the book.

   iii. Plan your eating times.
   Eat regularly through the day to ward off cravings for unhealthy food & stimulants.

   iv. Plan what you eat in advance.
   A good rule of thumb is to at least have a rough idea of what you'll eat for the next twenty-four hours. If you know good food

---

1   http://www.drugaddictiontreatment.com/drug-addiction-treatments/exercise-may-be-beneficial-for-overcoming-cocaine-addiction/

choices won't be available where you'll be, then plan ahead & take food with you. I'll guide you on what good food choices are later in this book.

v. *Make sure you are well nourished.*
Vitamin & mineral deficiencies can cause cravings. Having yearly or twice yearly full nutritional profiles completed could save you a lot of time, effort & pain. When your vitamin & mineral stores are at optimal you will recover quicker from exercise, suffer less injuries & illness plus experience less cravings.

vi. *Go to bed on time.*
Be conscious of the amount of rest you get. When you are tired, you'll crave stimulants to keep you going. The time you get to sleep is critical. How well you sleep & for how long is just as important.

vii. *Get into nature more.*
This could be as simple as a five-minute walk in the park or even just walking on grass, whatever is accessible. Try this barefoot. It will feel good because it will help relax reducing your cortisol output.

viii. *Drink more water.*
As soon as a craving arises, drink as much water as you can. You may find this extinguishes the craving for some time or altogether. Some cravings can be related to dehydration.

ix. *Use stimulants early in the day.*
Do not consume them after four thirty.

x. *Focus on the benefits.*
Have a clear picture of your goal. It may be better health, increased productivity, a better sex life, a six-pack & so on. In the moment of craving, get excited about your ultimate goal, whatever it is. This will help you stay on track.

xi. *Keep yourself busy.*

When cravings hit, apply yourself to a task & tell yourself that you'll complete it first & then maybe see to the craving. If the craving isn't as intense after completion of the task, forget about it.

xii. *Resist the craving for as long as possible.*

Sometimes a craving will be mild & easy to resist. Other times, it can be unbearable, relentless & continuous. Resist as long as you can. Each time the craving hits, stretch out how long you resist. Build up your resistance. Strengthen your willpower.

xiii. *Use teas.*

Herbal teas are great in moments of cravings. Get a selection; test which ones you like. Rotate them. Try new blends regularly. Drink these after four thirty rather than coffee. Be aware of herbal teas that contain caffeine, avoid these after four thirty.

xiv. *Breathe deeply.*

Before you give into a craving, take ten to twenty slow, deep, full breaths - Apply Principle 8. Then ask yourself can you resist for another five minutes. Keep increasing the period of resistance time. Once you begin to apply Principle 8 throughout your day automatically you will notice that many stressful situations do not have such an impact on you.

xv. *Supplement your sleep.*

This leads us to my next point…

4) Supplement your sleep

The time you go to sleep will affect your hormone levels, in particular growth hormone.

If you go to bed at a late hour every night, then you won't produce as much growth hormone as you would with a regular early night.

If your sleep is broken during the night, the production of growth hormone will also be interrupted. This is not a good thing.

When your production of growth hormone is inhibited, you will find it harder to increase lean muscle, recover from exercise & reduce body fat to name only a few related issues.

The human genome has not altered much in the past one hundred thousand years—approximately 1 percent. This means you function best when following the patterns of your ancestors—bringing us back to circadian rhythms.

The best time to get to sleep is at ten thirty pm.

From ten thirty pm until two am, your body focuses on physical repair.

From two until six in the morning, you benefit from mental & psychological repair.

Miss these time zones & you'll miss their benefits. If you wake up during these time zones, you'll interrupt & disrupt their full effects.

If you regularly go to sleep after ten thirty & suffer with regular physical injuries or complications, this is likely a root cause of your complaint(s).

The same goes for mental & psychological complications if you often wake during the two to six o'clock slot.

Manage these time frames better & notice the difference. It really is that simple. If you don't believe me, test it for yourself. You'll be amazed. I'll help you improve the quality of your sleep with suggestions & guidance; this will have a positive knock on affect throughout your life.

i. Water

As mentioned earlier as little as 2 percent dehydration will cause as much as a 30 percent drop in physical performance.

How does water affect your sleep? The answer is simple, "Give your body exactly what it needs & it will be healthy & function perfectly."

Give your body most of what it needs & it will be healthy most of the time & function as you want, some of the time. You get the point.

You are designed to be healthy. Full stop. If you're not at your best, or are ill or generally unhealthy, then I suggest that the cause is a lack of something specific. For now, take this point on board, as we'll continue to build on this theory as you read on.

Your body requires certain amounts of water in order to function optimally. Optimal intake of clean water is essential for detoxification & optimal function of your cells.

When you sleep, your body does many things, but the main two are detoxification & repair. If you are even slightly dehydrated of clean water, then your body's ability to detox will be slightly impaired. Majorly dehydrated = major impairment.

Drink adequate amounts of water throughout your day. Stop drinking water up to an hour before you go to bed. On rising, rehydrate yourself by drinking up to a pint of clean water. This will ensure that your body has what it needs when it needs it.

You'll notice less joint stiffness & pain; healthier, clearer hair, skin & nails; & a healthier shine to your eyes, to name but a few benefits from optimal water intake.

ii. Multivitamin

As mentioned, when you sleep, your body detoxes. Every toxin requires a certain vitamin or mineral to remove it from your body.

If you're deficient in a particular vitamin or mineral, then your detox process will be inhibited, as you simply do not have the raw material to mobilise & excrete the related toxin.

Your body won't allow this toxin to roam around your bloodstream. Instead, the toxin is stored in fatty tissue away from your internal organs—usually on your belly, hips, butt, or legs.

Every day, a number of toxins arrive, mostly from your environment. If you don't have the relevant vitamin or mineral, the same storage process is applied!

Can you see that if a person does not eat a healthy well balanced diet (or supplement) how it could be hard to decrease their body fat? Missing nutrients – inability to detox – increased fat storage… no matter how hard that person trains.

Remember near the beginning of this book I gave you the three main causes of obesity:

> i.   Toxicity
> ii. Stress
> iii. Malnutrition

Here we are talking about a form of malnutrition. You may have been shocked to see that as the third highest cause, but now you can begin to understand how this it is.

For a lot of people this is a root cause of stubborn body fat, inability to lose weight, lethargy & ill health.

One simple way to begin to combat this is by taking a quality multi-vitamin every day. I have sourced what I believe to be one of the best supplements on the market. You can get access to them through my website:

http://www.shapetrainer.co.uk/supplements.php

Try Multi Intense or Complete Multi.

iii. Magnesium

Talking about supplements, this is one of my favorites: magnesium.

Along with helping you get to sleep, keep you asleep & make sure you "sleep like a log," it's also involved in over three hundred cellular reactions within your body. It helps with muscle relaxation & reduces stress levels by calming your nervous system.

Magnesium is one of the most deficient minerals in the western world, especially in postmenopausal women. If you know people from this bracket, they have certainly told you about sleepless nights & muscle cramps.

This mineral can play a major role in improving your overall health not to mention your body composition. As mentioned previously, if your sleep is interrupted so will your ability to focus & perform at optimal. You will be acutely aware that when your sleep is negatively affected how that can negatively affect the rest of your life.

Your performance at work, in the gym or on the sports field will be hindered.

How much magnesium you should take depends on your personal status. The most accurate way to determine your levels is to have a red blood cell analysis. Then you can supplement according to your unique levels.

You should work with a professional to help you determine your current status & how to optimalise your vitamin & mineral levels.

The quality of the magnesium you use is also critically important. There are good brands & the opposite.

Again I have sourced one of the best magnesium supplements in the market. As there are 9 different forms of magnesium, & they all offer a different benefit to your body, it a good idea to rotate your magnesium supplement blends.

I suggest you work with a functional medicine doctor or medical professional to help you with this.

You can get access to top quality magnesium supplementation here:

http://www.shapetrainer.co.uk/supplements.php

Try UberMag PX or Zen Mag.

Chamomile tea

Chamomile tea is one of the most relaxing drinks to have before bed.

This tea has many properties that promote a better night's sleep. It is anti-inflammatory, antiseptic, carminative & sedative.

A lot of people drink sugary drinks or hot milk before bed. These beverages are stimulants & decrease your ability to relax & therefore sleep like a baby.

Eat your carbs at night

Eating carbohydrates at nighttime stimulates the release of tryptophan, which helps you sleep.

Tryptophan is an essential amino acid. It must be obtained from the diet & cannot be synthesised within the human body.

It is linked with serotonin, your happy neurotransmitter, which is why you may feel happier when you eat carbs. Basically put, increasing tryptophan brings about a relaxed, sleepy state. This is what you want later in your day!

On the flip side, what do you think eating carbs in the morning will do for you?

Inversely, eating protein in the morning will have the opposite effect—waking you up & making you feel alert & alive with an increased ability to concentrate. This happens through increasing production of dopamine – your neurotransmitter of attention & concentration.

Does the type of carbohydrate matter? For instance does it matter if you eat chocolate or sweet potato, or a piece of fruit? The answer is yes. The best choice of carb would be low GI. This stands for glycemic index. The lower the GI of the food the slower its energy is released into your blood stream

Further on I'll go in to more detail about GI & diet related info. I'll explain exactly what foods & when to eat them & go in to detail about what I have found to be a healthy balanced diet.

5) Harness the power of the dark

When you sleep, the room should be pitch black.

As mentioned, studies show that an LED light as small as a pin tip shone on the sole of your foot increases cortisol levels & pulls you out of deep sleep. This affects your ability to detox, repair cells & production of growth hormone.

Another issue with inconsistent sleep is that it interrupts your production of melatonin. The pineal gland produces melatonin, which is associated with sleep-wake cycles.

Melatonin production naturally decreases with age, but it can also be blocked, drained & nullified.

This affects sleep & long-term disruption has links with many health issues. Also associated with melatonin / sleep disruption are: irregular moods, reduced immune function, memory deficits, aging of the brain & body tissues, headaches, autism, cancer…this list goes on!

Obvious, but Often Missed

When our ancestors were cave people, they didn't use artificial light. When it became dark, they may have lit up their immediate surroundings with fire, but, soon after it became dark, they went to sleep.

The setting sun is a signal from nature that it's time to rest: physically, mentally & emotionally. When it starts to get dark outside it is a signal to you that you should begin to wind down for the day.

What happens if you don't follow this pattern? The truth is that you predispose yourself to illnesses & disease. I'm not saying that if you have a late night, you'll wake up with tuberculosis. What I am saying is that you increase your chances of getting a physical injury, picking up an illness & contracting a disease.

You also decrease your ability to perform at optimal.

If you do not follow this cycle it is just a matter of time before you start to feel your powers decreasing.

Embrace pitch-blackness.

Your bed is your private space. When you get into bed every night, ask yourself these two important questions:

1) Do I feel safe?
2) Do I feel comfortable?

If the answer to one or both of these questions is *no,* then you must address this *immediately.*

Do whatever is necessary to switch your mind off to possible dangers. Lock the doors. Get an alarm. Make sure your fire alarm system is fully functional. Solve whatever is on your mind so you can be at ease when your head hits the pillow.

This may require some mental management around your business or personal life. When you put your head on that pillow you must switch off. This is critically important to your long-term health & success.

If your bed is uncomfortable, it will disturb your sleep, impair your recovery & hinder you in more ways than are immediately apparent. Invest in the best bed that money can buy. In the long term it will be worth it.

Do whatever it takes to improve your sleeping conditions. This will benefit the rest of your life. Investing in the best bed you can afford is one of the wisest moves you can make.

If your bed doesn't engulf you into a deep, restful unconsciousness, then you need to understand why–& do something about it.

Like one of my clients said to me, "My bed swallows me up & spits me out in the morning. I'm totally gone in that time" This is the sleeping experience you are looking for – every night.

Principle Exercise 8
SSSSH Techniques

It is impossible to not be exposed to stress. So a smart decision would be to master techniques that manage stress well.

Optimal sleep is arguably your greatest ally.

From the previous chapters I have provided you detail about what an optimal sleep pattern should look & feel like:
Optimal Sleep times
Optimal Sleep duration
Optimal Sleep conditions
How to improve the quality of your sleep
How to supplement your sleep

Your exercise is to practice & combine all of the information above. At first it may seem like a lot but after a few applications the methods will start to become automatic.

Once this happens you notice a dramatic improvement throughout your waking day. Increased ability to focus, increased energy levels, increased stamina both mentally & physically, improved decision-making & the time it takes to make decisions in stressful situations will also decrease.

One Last Exercise: If all else fails then do this:

As you lie in bed, inhale & count one, exhale & count two. Inhale – one, exhale – two. Continue this sequence thinking of nothing else but these numbers.

This is a hypnotherapy technique that you can use on yourself. You will fall to sleep quicker & it will help switch your mind of so that you stay asleep longer & get a more restful nights sleep.

Principle 8
I Sleep Optimally Every Night.

For improved long-term health, there are few things better for your body

than deep, quality sleep.

Improving your sleep will improve your performance at work,

home & every other area of your life.

Quality sleep can have a profound impact on your memory & your ability to perform at a high level, both mentally & physically.

Provide the surroundings & complete the steps that ensure you get quality sleep every night. You will not regret it.

It's time to apply the techniques I just gave you in the last chapter.

Read them & attempt to apply as many of them as you can straight away.

Within the next seven days, make sure you are applying all of the SSSSH principles

When you begin to sleep optimally your energy & performance levels will go through the roof.

If you find it difficult to get to sleep or remain asleep throughout the night there is an issue that must be addressed as soon as possible.

The ideas I have provided you within this section will help. Apply all of them & give them at least two weeks to begin having affect.

You may need further support to perfect your sleep, which I will help you with as you read on.

Once you are applying all of the principle of Optimalism your sleep patterns will most definitely improve.

Now that we have completed an overview of optimal lifestyle habits, we can move on to your next step—exercise.

Solution 2: Exercise

Chapter 5:
Mechanics of Weight Training

Physical fitness is not only one of the most important keys to a healthy body; it is the basis of dynamic and creative intellectual activity.

—John F. Kennedy

Now that you have a firm grasp on your personal best lifestyle, it's time we move on to the exercise sections of Optimalism.

In this section, I present six main movements that I feel should be the core of your training programs.

An exercise program is only effective for as long as it takes for your body to adapt to it. This essentially means that you should alter your training routine every six workouts.

As a general rule of thumb it takes six workouts before a person begins to plateau for that routine. Therefore I suggest you alter your training sequence after six complete rotations.

Exercise positively affects your mental, emotional & physical state in a number of ways. It can boost happy moods, improve self-confidence, prevent cognitive decline, improve co-ordination through stimulation of the nervous system, alleviate anxiety, increase longevity & enhance productivity to name only a few benefits.

A moment spent on effective exercise is never wasted, as it enhances all forms of energy throughout your body.

Who wouldn't want these benefits? So what is it that usually stops people from making exercise a regular part of their life?

Within this section I aim to make exercise selection an easier process. I believe that the 6 main movements I will explain should be the staple of your workout routines.

As I will explain, these exercises are compound movements – require more than one joint to perform & therefore require a greater number of muscle fibres & motor neurons to be recruited.

Let's lunge into it…

Principle Exercise 9
Grow Inner Strength

Breathe deeply & then exhale.
As you exhale, contract your pelvic floor muscles.
These are the muscles you contract when you stop yourself
from urinating or prevent a bowel movement.

Not that we want to interrupt these natural processes but rather
strengthen the muscles involved with controlling them.

These are called kegal exercises. [1]

For practice create the feeling that you are pulling these muscles
up toward the center of your body.

Hold your breath for two seconds while strongly contracting these
muscles up & in.

Relax for two to five seconds & then repeat this movement five
to ten times.Completely relax these muscles in between each
contraction.

As a result of this exercise you will experience increased energy levels.
These types of exercises are used by yogis to build energy from within
their bodies. Yogis are yoga experts combining mediation & religion
as a practice as in Buddhism & Hinduism. They often also use tantric
sex practices to harness sexual energyfor greater health & vitality.

These exercises are used to return closer to optimal function of this
area of the body after prostrate cancer[2] Performing these exercises
could also stimulate greater health of the prostrate as men age.

---

1 http://urology.ucla.edu/body.cfm?id=408

2 http://www.theherald.com.au/story/2525555/mens-pelvic-floor-exercises-could-prevent-prostate-related-incontinence/

For women these muscles are important for managing incontinence & prolapse after childbirth. It is important to begin strengthening them as early as possible - even if you are not thinking of having children as this will help with bladder & bowel control.

Practice this movement daily to improve your internal & sexual energy levels.It works just as well for women as it does for men.

There are two main goals with this exercise:
1) To strengthen your deep internal muscles. These are good if you ever need to control the desire to urinate or have a bowel movement.

2) To bring a deeper focus to your breathing pattern. We will develop this as you read on. When combining the strength of these muscles & your breathing pattern we increase the support for your lower back, decreasing the chance of injury as your training routine increases in intensity & complexity.

Principle 9:
I Constantly Build Inner Strength.

Gain control of your inner strength. Build it up using the given exercise.

This helps stimulate greater health, vitality & sexual presence, Later we'll integrate this exercise into a weight-lifting technique that decreases the chances of you injuring your back.

Begin to think about where you can use this technique. If you've ever had a low back injury you can reduce your discomfort or eliminate pain. If you want to lift heavy in the gym you can integrate this into your lifting technique.

You can train these muscles anywhere at anytime. Become aware of how they work when you sit & stand, when you go to the bathroom & when you are exercising.

Believe me the stronger they are the healthier you will be. This is one little piece to the puzzle.

Remember - perfect practice makes perfect.

Want Heroic Results?

Resistance training, also called weight or strength training, encompasses a series of deliberate movements performed with weights to add "resistance" to your muscles.

These weights often come in the form of dumbbells, bars, cables, ropes, chains, or bands. Different responses are triggered in your body when you use these various loads to stimulate movement as you exercise.

The great thing about weight training is that progress can be never-ending, in the sense that you can keep progressing forever & keep learning new, improved ways to train that stimulate better performance & body composition.

This has been happening to me for years. It's a constant, evolving conversation between experts all over the world. A never-ending, forever evolving conversation packed with information & data about the human body & mind.

One main thing I have found over the years is that most people who lift weights do not adequately stimulate their muscular systems for maximum growth & response.

It's deceptively easy to spend weeks, even months, lifting—with little to no results. Don't fear; this section is designed to eradicate this possibility from your experience.

How Do You Choose to Look?

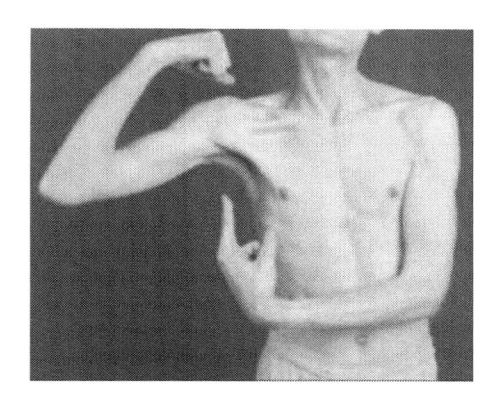 vs.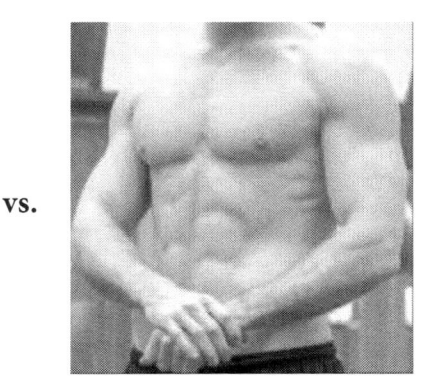

Good Free Weights Are Not Cheap

A quality set of free weights can set you back a tidy penny but they could last you a lifetime. So the investment could be well worth. Or you could just head down to your local gym, as long as the equipment there is what you are looking for.

Most commercial gyms are packed with cardio machines & lack a good free weight section. When selecting your gym make sure the free weight section has been paid a lot of attention.

Free-weight training is completed with dumbbells or a bar. The weight you choose determines the intensity of your workout & the eventual response you'll stimulate from your body.

Maintaining good posture while at the same time pushing your limits for each lift is the key to getting the most out of your workouts.

There are two main benefits with resistance training & thousands of secondary benefits:

1. Free-weight training translates into real-life fitness

Training at the gym with these movements with added weight will improve the movements you perform in daily life.

Squatting 20 kg (44lbs), for example, makes squatting without the weight feel easy. The more you practice, the easier & stronger these movements become.

An hour of this every day & the remaining twenty-three hours will feel like a soft summer breeze or walk in the park.

2. Fastest adaptations from your body

When you challenge your muscles to perform movements with added weight, muscle growth is stimulated & muscle tone naturally follows.

Weight "Focus"

Let's say you lay down, completely still, for twenty-four hours. Let's also say, for argument's sake, that you would burn five hundred calories to remain alive in that period of time, just for breathing & bodily functions.

If you participated in a seven-week intensive weight-training program, then lay back down for twenty-four hours, you would burn approximately, for argument's sake, 750 to 800 calories. That's an added 250 to 300 more calories—at rest. (Crude example but you get the point)

This extra calorie burn comes from the added muscle that you grew while working your muscles in this specific way. Picture muscles to be '*calorie furnaces*'. Fact is, the more lean muscle you have the more calories you will burn.

Imagine adding movement to the example above. You will double or quadruple your energy expenditure – per day.

It's a crude example, but the point is that caloric expenditure rapidly increases when you focus on weight training.

The more muscle you have, the more calories (fat or energy) you burn. A great weight-training program will make your body burn fat like crazy, with no diet change at all. Then if you improve your diet, you would get even better results.

More muscle also means more efficient use of energy & fat. Business people who are serious about getting in shape should use free weights when training. Sports professionals who are not yet benefitting from strength training (weight training) sessions should start immediately as they will have not reached their full potential.

This type of training offers instant results & has far-reaching long-term benefits.

The Gym Machine

Every modern gym should have easy-to-use weight machines. They exist so that you can incorporate them into your weight-training program to build muscle—easy. Weight machines can be an added tool for you while at the gym.

These are the large, heavy machines people use to push, pull, or twist through any number of specific targeted movements. All you do is add weight, move & resist that weight in certain directions or ranges of motion.

Often you need to sit, stand, or bend in a particular way when you use these machines so that you can focus on one specific muscle group. Or even target a muscle in a specific way.

Machine weights were originally created to facilitate postural habilitation. Physiotherapists could target specific muscles through safe ranges of motion after surgery or injury to a joint, muscle, or bone.

Body builders adopted them after their success in strengthening weak or injured body parts. They are a great way to pinpoint & sculpt specific muscle groups—ideal when developing the perfect physique.

The average person, however, (someone who is not injured & is not a body builder) will not require them on a regular basis.

They should be sprinkled into a training program, unless you are suffering from an injury, when they will be the core of your training routine, or a body builder where you may utilise their ability to pinpoint muscle fibers.

Movement in everyday life is in 3D—there is no support, no controlled direction & range of motion is specific to your joint. Weight machines are great, but they should take up on average no more than 10 percent of your training program.

Machines are not the main way you should train your body & muscles every day. Free weights are far more effective. Overuse of weight machines does not help you build supporting musculature or the stabilizer muscles that literally stabilize your spine & joints.

Without free movement, you do not effectively stimulate these muscle groups, which can leave your core & joints weak, as well as predispose you to injury.

These core stabilizer muscles are important to overall health & injury prevention. Movement in 3D needs to be a part of a balanced health & fitness-training program.

Machines Can Benefit You. . .One Hot Tip

If you like hitting the gym, then you may have access to weight machines more often than most people do. Under certain circumstances, weight machines *do* have a solid place in a quality training program.

As mentioned, injured individuals, postoperative strength trainers & body builders benefit the most from weight machines. A select few machines, if used intermittently, will benefit the average person.

The majority of your weight training should mimic real life. Machines are not the most effective means of achieving this carryover. But they can help you work on any problem areas you may have.

You can achieve a better looking, more functional body by training predominantly with free weights in comparison to machine workouts.

If you use machines sparingly, your joints & long-term fitness will benefit. Mix them in with free weights for maximum muscle gain, nervous system stimulation & continual improvement.

There may be compelling reasons to avoid weight machines altogether. I have never met a novice gym user who knows how to safely & efficiently use free weights—which adds to the problem of machine weight overuse.

The solution is to train with a regular gym goer who knows how to use free weights properly, or hire an expert to teach you the right moves.

It helps if the expert actually knows how to use free weights in an effective way.

Machines May Not Be the Answer

If you want to be a monster body builder like Arnie, then, sure, focus on *combining* free-weight training with machines.

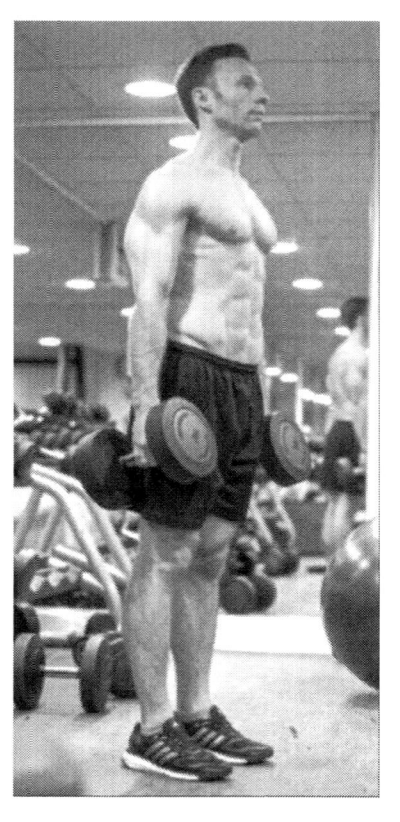

Please be aware that many gym-offered training programs are run by young people fresh off the press (recently completed their qualifications). They may have great energy, but they do not have the experience or practical understanding to train you safely yet. Always be cautious.

The question of who uses weight machines the most is worth exploring.

Look around the next time you're at the gym; Who looks the fittest?

Who looks healthiest?

Who has the highest percentage of body fat?

Who looks older?

You'll notice that, on average, the people in the free weight section look the least stressed, have the biggest muscles & have the lowest percentage of body fat.

This will give you insight into your own training & where you should spend most of your time in the gym.

Or if you find that after a few months of using free weights, you'd like to "polish" the look of certain muscles or add variation to your routine by using weight machines, then fine.

There's a real difference between looking fit & actually being fit. The obvious difference is that people who look fit do not necessarily have the health benefits that an authentically fit person has. That is what you want.

The most intelligent thing you can do is get a coach. There are many intricacies involved in a comprehensive training program, especially if you are after results that last.

Lifting weights kills fat; that is a fact. To lose fat, live longer, become more attractive & enjoy a more active life, lift free weights.

Weight Lifting versus Cardio: The Battle

Weight training is the key to low body fat percentage, living longer, feeling strong inside & looking strong from the outside.

That doesn't mean that cardio training has no place in your program. Certain types of cardio exercises are more effective for reducing belly fat & increasing your fitness levels quickly, especially if you have defined goals.

Why do I prefer weights to cardio? A few reasons:

- *Cardio makes you look older.*
  Engaging in long bouts of cardiovascular training, for example long-distance running, stimulates increased insulin. In the long-term, higher insulin secretion

will age your cells & make you appear older than you really are.

- **Weight training makes you look younger.**
  Aside from looking more toned & muscular, which is naturally youthful, regular weight training improves your insulin sensitivity & helps you combat the effects of excessive insulin in your cells.[1]

- **Cardio increases oxidative stress.**
  Weight lifting reduces it. Oxidative stress happens when there is an oxygen imbalance in your body & you are unable to adequately or quickly repair the resulting damage. Long bouts of cardio can promote this effect. Some effects of oxidative stress are Neurodegenerative disorders such as Parkinson's disease, multiple sclerosis & Alzheimer's, Cancer, heart attacks, Chronic fatigue syndrome, Diabetes, Gut disorders such as inflammatory bowel disease to name only a few. This can be reduced by altering your training & managed by improving your antioxidant intake through your diet.

- **Cardio decreases longevity.**
  Weight lifting increases longevity by improving a number of specific variables related to aging[2]. Surprising as it sounds, extreme cardio can actually reduce your life expectancy[3]. Studies have highlighted that moderate cardio training is optimal for longevity & health. The amount required for optimal health is unique to each individual & their circumstances. I suggest that within this optimal amount that there is

---

1 http://care.diabetesjournals.org/content/21/8/1353.abstract

2 *http://www.cdc.gov/physicalactivity/growingstronger/why/*

3 http://www.ncbi.nlm.nih.gov/pmc/articles/PMC3538475/

also an optimal approach – the type of cardio exercise is also critical. More about this later.

- ***Long bouts of Cardio are time consuming.***
  Weight lifting brings about immediate noticeable adaptations where as cardio is looked upon as more of an internal improvement. But can you gain the same internal benefits you get from cardio workouts from weight training workouts? Absolutely. The type of weight training exercises that you perform is critical just like the type of cardio exercises you choose. You may at present run many miles per week without seeing the physical change you want. As explained earlier, weight training burns more calories throughout the day. You will grow more muscle & burn more fat in half the time—which will keep you motivated.

- ***Cardio workouts are predominantly lower body focused.***
  With weight training workouts, you can target any area or specific muscle of your body. Overall lean muscle mass is much more important for lowering disease risk, improving fitness levels, increasing energy levels & increasing lifespan—all while burning more fat. It is important to live with balance particularly throughout the structure of your body. When out of balance you will likely experience pain – for instance muscular imbalance can cause joint pain or injury. Postural imbalance can cause pain & discomfort that continues throughout your day. With weight training & resistance exercises you can balance your muscular system & eliminate imbalance, therefore reducing your stress load through reducing stress on your joints & body.

Chapter 6:
The Vitality in
Cardiovascular Training

"If I could only do one exercise, it would be dead lifting. For cardio, I dance, I ride my bike, I run and I have kids. There is a... lot of cardio just from being a parent".

- Hugh Jackman

Most people expect vast amounts of cardiovascular exercise when they start a new training program. Running, cycling, aerobics appear to the average person like the most logical thing to do. More movement must mean more calories burnt right - basically it does. However, there is more going on within the optimal health & fitness puzzle than just that.

This logical thought process holds some truth but is it the most effective use of your time? Are there movements that you can perform that will bring about better results for your time spent & greater health benefits? Are some forms of cardiovascular training more effective than others?

The general understanding & approach to health & fitness is obviously not working. Western societies are getting fatter even though the cardio equipment is getting more sophisticated.

There is a more effective approach that you can take. I'll talk you through a different structure to what the average person is doing. I'll show you ways to train that have been working extremely well for some while others slave away on treadmills & bikes for hours on end.

Are long bouts of cardio lasting over an hour the most health promoting, time efficient & most effective forms of exercise? Definitely not!

Do You Know?

Cardio training is supposed to challenge your cardiovascular system— your heart, blood vessels & lungs. Obvious right. It is quite literally the way blood travels through your body.

The healthier you are, the less resistance there is to blood reaching all areas of your body. When you work out, your heart pumps harder & circulates blood faster. This type of training can & does, strengthen your heart.

Your cardio system also uses your lungs, because blood needs to be oxygenated. Increasing demand of blood to your muscles requires more blood oxygenation—which is why you breathe harder when you exercise.

Naturally, cardio training is good for you—but are long bouts of cardio the smartest choice for optimal health, fitness & body composition?

My answer to you is no, not really. Not if you're looking to live longer, decrease your body fat stores, manage your weight & keep the chance of injury to a minimum.

It appears that people love to pound away on treadmills, rowers & bikes to burn energy & lose fat. After fifteen years in the industry & hundreds of trained clients—not to mention the scientific evidence—I have to say that more than one hour of cardio every day is wrong.

Working out for more than an hour at a time will stress your body & raise your cortisol levels – stress hormone. This will lead to difficulty reducing fat around your umbilicus (belly button) as well a number of other issues.

Cardio workouts which usually last between 20 minutes to over an hour will eventually contribute to aging you before your time!—thanks to consistently raised insulin levels.

Remember, insulin ages your cells & prolonged bouts of cardiovascular training on a regular basis has proven to raise insulin levels.[1]

Rampant Insulin stimulated through specific diet & training regimes will harm you rather than help you.

Certain types of cardio can be enormously beneficial, Anaerobic workouts – sprint or high intensity interval training (HIIT) have proven to drop fat stores, improve blood pressure & increase insulin sensitivity (a good thing) more than steady state cardio sessions. This is to name only a few benefits.[2]

Think of a sport like football or soccer. Most would look at the sport & think that it requires considerable cardiovascular endurance or the ability to run long distance – but on closer examination from motion capture analysis it highlights that it is in fact a game of repeated sprints.

The ability to repeat sprints & repeat them while under fatigue is far more specific to this sport.[3]

---

1 http://bjsm.bmj.com/content/44/Suppl_1/i17.4.abstract

2 http://www.ncbi.nlm.nih.gov/pubmed/8028502

3 file:///Users/danielgrant/Downloads/The%20role%20and%20development%20of%20sprinting%20speed%20in%20soccer.pdf

It has been shown in many studies that anaerobic workouts are far more effective at reducing body fat, alongside many other health benefits.[4]

One such study published in the journal of obesity shows that high intensity exercise increases both anaerobic & aerobic fitness, significantly lowers insulin resistance & results in increases in skeletal muscle capacity for fatty acid oxidation & glycolytic enzyme content - all good stuff by the way.[5]

The point being that choosing your cardio workouts wisely will lead to a more successful response from the time spent working out; increased health benefits, improved body composition, improved health status alongside the all important matter of saving you time!

Think of it like this - you wake up, you're extremely busy all day until you chase yourself into bed at night. Adding long bouts of cardio to this lifestyle pattern will not help you. Whereas a few short sprints at maximal or sub-maximal pace will serve you better for optimal body composition, health & performance.

A Short Cardio Theory

You don't have to stop all cardio training. In small amounts, cardio can & is, essential to a healthy body & mind.

Long-distance running, long-duration cardio training of over one hour at a time can be detrimental to your health. Look around, the world is getting fatter, not thinner. In the most part people's lives are also getting busier.

If cardio burned fat so well, why are most people that you see in the cardio sections at the gym still fat?

4 http://www.ncbi.nlm.nih.gov/pmc/articles/PMC2991639/

5 http://www.ncbi.nlm.nih.gov/pmc/articles/PMC2991639/

There is a real disconnect here. Surely lots of cardio would ensure that super-busy individuals like you would be in tip-top shape? Nope. Perhaps fewer people go to the gym, or they all have bad diets & too much stress in their lives. This is likely.

Let me put it this way. Millions of people do cardio every day & stay fat. Very few people partake in a well-designed resistance-training program & that is one big reason why they remain fat.

Overall a well-structured resistance-training program offers many of the same health adaptations as cardiovascular training with additional benefits also.

In fact, as a lifestyle, weight training is far more effective & time efficient in comparison to long bouts of cardiovascular exercise. One of these studies from the University of Calgary looked at the effects of aerobic, resistance & a combination of the two.[1]

Results showed that resistance training was the most effective form of exercise for fat loss & improvement in cardiometabolic risk markers.

Why do so many people still hit the pavement or the parks, running for up to an hour or in some cases more?

There is a real lack of access to accurate information in the world, even with the Internet available to most of us. There is no shortage of information—but out of all that information what is accurate or true & what is false?

With the Internet, incorrect information can spread like wildfire. Just because something is a popular opinion does not mean it is right, or the only way to reach optimal health or fitness.

1 http://www.ncbi.nlm.nih.gov/pubmed/25243536

Short-burst cardio is worth engaging in. As you are not just about working hard, you are about working smart, this type of cardio is your wisest choice. For a person who is highly successful & wants results quickly interval training is the way to go.

Leave the long-distance cardio to specific endurance event training. If you don't participate in these types of sport then do not stress your system with long cardio sessions.

For your cardio workouts you will get better results & save a lot of time by following the guidelines I provide you here. I'll present some more details around the facts I have presented in a moment.

You can gain all the benefits, the mental clarity & endorphin rush from a quality resistance-training program. One study from the center for sports medicine at Pennsylvania State University showed that testosterone, growth hormone & cortisol are all elevated by resistance training exercise.

In fact it showed that the more experienced weight lifters had greater effects on these hormones. Indicating that regular resistance training positively stimulates these hormones, therefore providing the 'exercise rush' that so many people love.[1]

Obviously if you participate in marathons, or long distance sports then you must train specifically for that sport. The point being here that for nearly everything else including 'everyday' health & fitness then interval training is a smarter choice.

Also, you may find improved performance from phasing in some interval training into your program even if it is long distance sports you regularly partake in.

---

1 http://www.ncbi.nlm.nih.gov/pubmed/1555898

It will challenge your system in an alternative way & allow areas of your body to recover in preparation for continued long distance work in the near future.

Interval Training Explained

You can achieve a quicker drop in body-fat & increases in sports performance from interval training, which is still a subset of cardiovascular exercise. You perform the same movement at varying speeds. This encourages the energy systems in your body to work at different times & for different durations – they way they are supposed to work.

You walk, jog & sprint intermittently for periods of time. You rarely need more than thirty minutes. You don't need to take an entire hour at the gym, solely for cardio.

Fat-loss experts commonly recommend twenty-minute bursts of interval training, combined with a good weight-training program.

When you focus on interval training, you don't exhaust any of your systems for prolonged periods of time. Your whole body is used—internally your heart, lungs & circulatory system & also your muscular systems are challenged in a positive way.

Sprint intervals are my favorite cardio exercise. They involve a small warm-up, followed by repeated sets of fast paced movement (a sprint) separated by a recovery period. The length of the sprint & recovery period is determined by the energy system that you want to focus on & your goal.

You can also adjust the number of sets (number of sprints) that you perform depending on specific requirements.

The sprint works you anaerobically—without oxygen—so you stimulate your anaerobic energy system, which is different from the one you use when walking or jogging (aerobic energy system – with oxygen).

When oxygen demand is greater than supply, your anaerobic energy system takes over. Think of the physical appearance of Olympic sprinters & world champion long-distance runners. Sprinters use the anaerobic energy system & distance runners use the aerobic energy system.

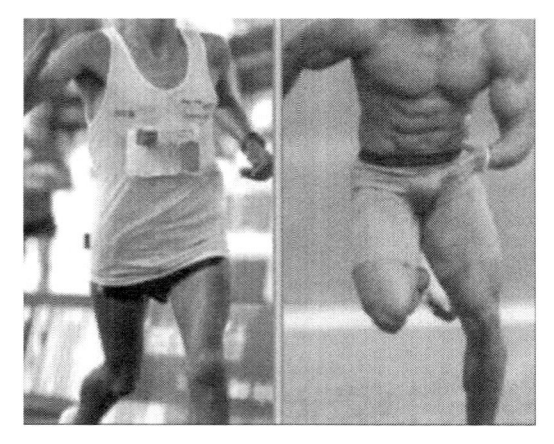

One stimulates muscle growth, the other burns fat *& muscle!* That is why sprinters are stacked with muscle plus remain low body-fat & long-distance runners look thin but at the same time carry little muscle mass.

Both sports produce low body-fat. However if you want more muscle definition then get into sprint training as your form of cardio workout.

The more muscle you have, the more calories you burn. It really is that simple. It's one thing to look lean, but having to run for over an hour every day to maintain it is another, then you must wonder if that type of training is supporting optimal health & fitness overall.

Forty-five to sixty minutes of weight training, combined with sprints three times per week will bring you good results for fat loss & a toned, muscular look.

I have achieved excellent results from interval training & I have cut people's cardio workout times in half, while getting them to double their muscle tone & drop body-fat. Success!

Call me nuts, but if I want to burn fat, I want to know the most efficient way to get this done, as soon as possible - rather than wasting my time with exercises that bring very little to no change on my physique & health.

That means maximum calorie burn in the shortest space of time. That means the more muscle available the easier I achieve this goal.

I don't have time to waste & I assume you don't either.

An Example Sprint Session:

- Choose a piece of equipment or go outside.

- Start your movement: treadmill, bike, outside running—whatever.

- Start slow; ease into the movement for two minutes, slowly picking up the pace.

- At two minutes, sprint.

- Full-out maximum effort for thirty seconds.

- At two minutes, thirty seconds, return back to your slow, steady pace. This is your active recovery period, for this example it lasts for one minute.

- Complete five sets of thirty second sprints, each followed by one minute moving recovery periods

- End with two to five minutes at a slow, steady pace as a warm-down & then perform some light stretches.

You can build up your number of sprints over time. As a general rule of thumb, look to increase one set of sprints every one to two weeks. Build yourself up to at least 10 sprints per session.

Principle Exercise 10
Nose Breathing

It may sound unusual to be given breathing exercises but the truth is that many people do not breath optimally, have weak breathing patterns & suffer in health or performance because of it.

Doctor Buteyko said "To be healthy you need to breathe properly". His method has been developed over 40 years & highlights the importance of optimal breathing.[1]

A technique used by rowers to improve their performance & finish to a race involves keeping their mouth closed & breathing just through their nose for the first three quarters of the race or training phase. Then toward the end they open the mouth & are able to uptake more oxygen, which helps for a faster finish.

When you are training at high intensity like the sprint session I suggested, your body requires more oxygen. By breathing through your nose you slightly restrict access to larger amounts of oxygen.

This causes the body to get used to working under stress while receiving less oxygen, improving the efficiency of oxygen & energy distribution throughout your body.

It also increases the strength of your breathing pattern, your breathing muscles, as your body fights to pull more air in.

Toward the end of the race or training period, when you want a sprint finish or you are making a final push to win the race, you open your mouth & intake large volumes of air, oxygenating your blood & providing you with a welcomed energy boost at the right time.

---

1 http://www.buteyko.co.uk/what-is-buteyko.htm

Principle 10:
I Strengthen My Breathing Pattern With Every Conscious Breath

You can use this technique when you are training or simple going about your day.

Breathe only through your nose for periods of time, feeling your breath rate increase & making your cardiovascular system work harder for periods of time.

Breathing through your nose tends to elongate your breath & encourages more use & expansion of your lungs.

After a period of time with closed mouth & nose breathing open your mouth & allow more air to enter your system.

You can also apply this to everyday movements. For example, a set of stairs, simply only breathe through your nose for the entire flight, near the top or after you reach the top open your mouth & breath deeply to recover.

Cardio is better optimised when you use this breathing technique intermittently to strengthen your breathing pattern.

A different area of your lungs will respond & you will receive a burst of energy when you open your mouth, which will stimulate higher performance levels & even greater clarity in your mind.

Simply by altering the way you breathe during a cardio workout or throughout your day, you can maximize the training that you are doing but consciously strengthening the muscles involved with breathing. This is how you also work smart with cardio.

No need for a two-hour run. You can have more physiological response from your body in half the time.

From Principle 8 you should already be aware of your breathing pattern & notice it throughout your day. As you have strengthened your optimal breathing pattern it is now time to take that strength into performance & train it there.

Use your breathing to help you, use your breathing as a support for optimal health, fitness & performance.

The Importance of Pelvic Power

The pelvic floor is an area of muscle & connective tissue that spans the area underneath the pelvis, separating the pelvic cavity above from the perineal region below. It provides support to the pelvic viscera including the bladder, intestines & uterus (in females).

It also assists with continence through control of the urinary and anal sphincters. Finally, it helps to maintain optimal intra-abdominal pressure[1]

These muscles & the system they are part of are often overlooked & undertrained.

They act in part, like a sling that supports your bladder & urethra (the tube that transports urine outside of the body).

The pelvic floor gives you greater control when urinating because it works synergistically with your bladder, allowing flow, or non-flow, of urine. The more you train your pelvic floor muscles, the easier it will be to control the flow of your urine.

Older adults will appreciate this advice. If you don't train these muscles regularly or restore them after giving birth for women, you will likely suffer with complications when going to the toilet later in life.

These issues include the inability to control urination, "pressure" urine leaking, problems emptying urine, accidental wind passing & prolapse (a bulging of one or more of the pelvic organs). This can occasionally lead to pain when having sex.

Weak pelvic floor muscles can contribute to the experience of back pain. I have worked with dozens of people who have completely

---

1 http://www.physio-pedia.com/Pelvic_Floor_Anatomy

resolved their back issues after strengthening their pelvic floor in combination with specific techniques to increase intra abdominal pressure & a postural strength program. More about this in a moment.

Increasing strength in this area & integrating that strength into regular movement patterns reverses the issues that are caused by weak pelvic floor muscles, reduces back pain & the occurrence of back injuries.

One study from the University of Queensland showed that strengthening the multifidus, transverse abdominus & pelvic floor muscles in a pre-determined exercise program decreased back pain for elite cricketers.[2]

The multifidus functions together with transverse abdominus & pelvic floor muscles to stabilise the low back & pelvis before movement of the arms & or legs occurs.

The transverse abdominus is a deep core muscle of your trunk. It aids in supporting your spine & internal organs when moving & when functioning optimally should contract before any movement of your arms or legs.

Why bother talking about this?

If you're going to reach your peak performance levels training your pelvic floor muscles will need to be a little task on the agenda.

It will support the long-term health of your bowels, strengthen your back through intra-abdominal pressure & can lead to heightened sexual experiences.

Intra abdominal pressure is the positive pressure that you can consciously put in place before any heavy lift or strenuous movement. It

---

2 http://www.ncbi.nlm.nih.gov/pubmed/18349481

will strengthen your trunk & support your spine. More about this in a moment.

An important point I want to stress is the strengthening of your back. Strengthening your pelvic floor muscles increases in support for your back. What this process does effectively is provide your back support that allows you to lift heavier (more) weight while decreasing the risk of back injury.

The more weight you lift & more repetitions you perform, the stronger & fitter you'll become.

The stronger & fitter you become, the more muscle you'll grow. The more muscle you grow the more calories you burn. The more calories you burn, the less likely you will get fat—ever.

Who wouldn't want these results?

Once you take yourself to your physical peak, you'll reach a plateau. This is true for everybody. There are subtle techniques that will blast you through your sticking points & keep you progressing.

Strong pelvic floor muscles, integrated into your lifting, are one of those techniques. They will not only provide you with greater lifting strength & power, they will also dramatically reduce your risk of injury, particularly to your lower back.

The longer you can train without a break or hindrance, the more of a steady upward progression you will experience.

As you can begin to see, these exercises are clearly worth the time & effort.

Intra-Abdominal Pressure: The Truth

This is something a lot of trainers don't talk about at all. Either they don't think it's important, or they don't know about it.

Intra-abdominal pressure can build within the trunk of your body. It supports your internal organs & spine, which, as you are now aware can make a big difference over time to your training loads & schedule.

Learning how to control this pressure involves strength training specific muscle areas to maintain pressure.

This decreases the load on your spine & has many other far-reaching benefits for overall health & wellness.

When you learn to control intra-abdominal pressure you:

- Decrease your chances of ever injuring your spine.

- Increase your chances of being able to lift more weight - safely.

- Improve your lifting technique.

- Increase your strength through proper technique

When you can decrease the chance of spinal injury & increase weight tolerance, you'll likely never be stopped due to back injury.

Consistent training sessions are the essence of what creates real results. To get the body you really want will take daily commitment & consistency—so injuries are a concern. That's why I focus on strengthening your ability to control intra-abdominal pressure.

An effective body is an injury-free body. The only way to keep an effective body functioning is to look after it.

Isolate, Then Integrate

The way to strengthen your pelvic floor is to first perform isolation exercises that focus only on those muscles. Then integrate that focus & strength into a lift or specific movement.

A book that provides a number of useful exercises to strengthen a part of this system, alongside some insightful tips for the bedroom is The Multi Orgasmic Man by Mantak Chia.

He explains that by cultivating your sexual energy you not only gain better control in the bedroom but also boost your immune system. On top of this, I am saying that you also strengthen your core & lower back.

Worth a little time & effort to develop this area of yourself I'm sure you'll agree.

The full technique, using all the muscles involved & a specific breath pattern is called thoracolumbar fascia gain.

This basically means you have positive tension across your midsection that supports your lower back.

It's simple once you know what you are doing.

Let's build this up a little more so you understand it.

Principle Exercise 11
Perfect Pelvic Pulsing

Part 1: Long Holds

- *Sit upright. Make sure your legs aren't crossed.*

- *Take a breath in.*

- *As you breathe out, contract the front area of your pelvic floor. This is the same muscle you use when you stop the flow of urine midstream.*

- *You can also practice this the next time you urinate. Allow it to flow, then stop the flow by contracting these muscles & then relax & allow it to flow again. Do this several times each time you urinate.*

- *Contract the muscles at the front. Draw that feeling up toward the center of your body behind your belly button & hold.*

- *Now contract the muscles at the back, in your rectum. You use these muscles when you restrict a bowel movement.*

- *Having contracted both sets of muscles, focus on drawing them up behind your belly button toward the center of your body. Do this as intensely as possible.*

- *Hold this contraction for five to thirty seconds. Start small & build up the duration of your hold over time. You should start to feel more & more aware of this muscle as it gets stronger. You'll feel that you can contract the muscle more intensely.*

• ***After each contraction, fully relax.*** *Create a feeling of pushing down & out as you relax to make sure these muscles switch off.*

• *The idea is to strengthen your "long-hold contraction" of these muscles. This gives you greater control of urination & provides you with increased resistance when the desire to urinate cannot be released, such as when you're sitting on a train or on a long drive, busting to go to the bathroom but still have a fifteen-minute ride ahead of you!*

• *These muscles will increase core endurance – your ability to hold a challenged position when exercising or playing a sport, which in turn can improve your performance.*

Part 2: Short Holds

The second way to condition this muscle group is through quick, short holds.

This is useful for powerful movements & sporting situations.

Your pelvic floor should contract 0.01 second before the movement of a limb.

So basically these deep muscles should switch on just before you move your arm or leg. They stabilise your core & protect your spine.

• *Use the same position as before.*

• *Rather than slowly drawing the muscles in, contract them both as quickly & as fully as possible. Focus on snapping them into their fully contracted position & hold for one second.*

- *Fully relax, pushing them out in the opposite direction for two seconds.*

- *Repeat this for twenty repetitions.*

- *With this exercise, you'll likely see movement in your abdomen.*

- *Work these muscles, not to total fatigue, but so that you are more aware of them. Feel like you've trained them, but not drained them.*

Principle 11
I Consciously Use Core Strength

A great thing about these exercises is that you can do them anywhere, anytime. No one can tell you're doing them (unless you pull a funny face while performing the contraction—which isn't necessary, by the way).

So practice daily & regularly, while sitting in your car, on the train, in a meeting,

urinating & so on.

Build up to thirty-second holds, rest for ten to fifteen seconds & repeat. Do this ten to fifteen times.

This means ten to fifteen sets of thirty-second holds, with ten- to fifteen-second rest periods between sets.

You can then follow this with twenty quick contractions,

or split the workouts up & alternate them throughout your day.

Once you have the hang of contracting this muscle intensely, practice the hold in different positions—for example, while standing, kneeling, bending over to pick something up, etc.

The idea is for you to be able to contract this muscle in any position you find yourself & feel strong & able. The better you get at this, the less chance you'll injure your back.

Remember practice does not make perfect...
Perfect practice makes perfect.

Another Muscle

The muscle that completes the protective cylinder for your spine that we are strengthening is the transverse abdominis.

This muscle is the deepest of your abdominal muscles. It wraps around your abdomen between the lower ribs & the top of your pelvis. Think of it like a corset that you can control to squeeze your trunk & hold your spine in a safe place.

It's the muscle that contracts when you stand side-on in the mirror & pull your belly in—yes, we've all done it!

The combination of your diaphragm, transverse abdominis & pelvic floor muscles make up this central spine-supporting cylinder.

Working Your Transverse

Think of pulling on a tight pair of pants. As you pull them up, you automatically pull your belly button toward your spine.

This works your transverse abdominis muscle. Strengthen this muscle in the same way as your pelvic floor—long contraction holds & short contraction holds. Apply the same exercises.

Practice the long & short holds, increasing your strength over time.

Principle Exercise 12:
Get Yourself Together

Integration

Now that you understand how to work these muscles in isolation, it's time to work them in unison with other areas of your body.

- *Take a deep breath in.*

- *As you exhale, contract your pelvic floor & transverse abdominis muscles at the same time. Hold them.*

- *While keeping them contracted, continue to breathe in & out.*

- *Contract these muscles as intensely as you can for ten full breaths.*

- *You'll increase the stamina of this system, which is essential for obtaining the full benefits.*

When lifting...

Let's integrate these techniques into your lifting patterns.

Before you squat, deadlift, bench press, or perform any major training movement, it's important that you activate thoraco-lumbar fascia gain or intra abdominal pressure (IAP) as explained above.

IAP is the full combination of a deep diaphragmatic breath bringing your diaphragm into place as the ceiling, contraction of your pelvic floor muscles bringing the floor into place & contraction of your transverse abdominus bringing the walls into place – the combination of these movements creates the support cylinder for your trunk & spine.

Over time & with a little practice, this will become automatic & will give you greater core stability, increase the strength of your lifts & decrease the risk of injury to your back

Set the tension within your trunk by applying the movements listed above – at this point hold a deep breath in.

Only when you have all these components in place do you move the weight.

Do this for every rep of every set.

Essentially, these specific internal movements are your bodies own weight belt. Think of weight lifters wearing those thick leather belts who can lift ridiculously heavy weights.

This is the same concept, but rather than the belt doing the work, your body's own weight belt performs the hold for you.

Your internal weight belt needs to be as strong as possible, for obvious reasons. Repeated use of an external weight belt triggers faulty recruitment patterns in your abdominal wall where you push your abdomen against the belt to brace your spine rather than pulling in to stabilise.[1]

The use of a weight belt has shown to minimally reduce the risk of injury.
Fact is that you're not going to wear one of these all the time & over time they create a faulty recruitment pattern leaving you at greater risk, on top of which studies have shown the benefits of a weight

---

1 http://www.ncbi.nlm.nih.gov/pubmed/10552322

belt are minimal when supporting the trunk when a sudden load is applied.[2, 3, 4]

Point being, strengthen & control your own weight belt through every movement & lift that compromises the integrity of your spine or lower back.

If you're a power lifter or avid weight lifter, intermittent use of an external weight belt can allow you to increase loads for certain lifts possibly stimulating progression or break in a plateau.

2 http://www.ncbi.nlm.nih.gov/pubmed/2141312

3 http://www.ncbi.nlm.nih.gov/pubmed/7709282

4 http://www.ncbi.nlm.nih.gov/pubmed/10774136

Principle 12
I Use Internal Pressure Wisely

Putting all of this together means you reduce the likelihood of injury to your lumbar spine (low back).

The technical name for this is thoracolumbar fascia gain, or intra abdominal pressure (IAP).

This basically means the coordinated contraction of these specific muscles, in combination with an inhalation at a specific time. Remember, your breath is part of this sequence.

Every time you lift something heavy (or anything over one kilogram), make sure you use this technique.

Over time, it will become automatic.

This sounds subtle, but, when used effectively, it can dramatically reduce your exposure to injury & the potential onset of back pain.

Having strength within these muscles as we get older has shown to reduce erectile dysfunction & postoperative prostrate issues for men[1] & support optimal urinary flow & control for women after pregnancy[2]

---

1 http://www.ncbi.nlm.nih.gov/pubmed/22573231

2 http://www.ncbi.nlm.nih.gov/pubmed/25648223

Chapter 7:
The Sport of Human Movement

Exercise to stimulate, not to annihilate. The world wasn't formed in a day, and neither were we. Set small goals and build upon them.

—Lee Haney

It's no secret that specific movement promotes life. It's been a well-known fact since the days of ancient Greece.

It's also why people feel a need to compete with each other, in order to keep pushing the boundaries of what is possible & evolving as physical beings.

The Olympics was one of the earliest forms of sport. By picking a sport you truly enjoy, you can support your daily exercise routine & contribute to your mental, emotional & psychological wellness—all at the same time.

How Sport Makes You Extra Fit

Fitness, as mentioned, is so much more than simply looking fit or even feeling physically able to take on challenging tasks. Health is another aspect entirely – not separate to, but containing its own requirements in order to be at optimal.

A person can be physically fit but not healthy. However when you combine the two you reach an optimal state of being.

Sport makes you extra fit, not just because it tones your muscles or gives you a good cardio workout (depending on the sport), but because it stimulates competition, motivation & inspires social engagement, which reduces stress, anxiety & worry.

So pick a sport you enjoy & do it at least once a week.

Here's how to select a sport that appeals to you:

- Which sports immediately catch your eye?

- Which sport did you enjoy as a kid?

- Do you have an existing passion for a particular sport?

- Do you currently have enough energy to play this sport?

- Does it stimulate you physically & mentally?

- Do you feel a burning desire to do well at this sport?

- Do you prefer the team or individual element of this sport?

- Do you have a friend or friends that paly a particular sport that you could join?

There are lots of sports to choose from. Pick one & make it a hobby of yours. It will enrich your life, expand your overall fitness & lead to great health & wellness in the long run.

Master of Movement that Matters

Which movements provide you with the most bang for your buck in regards to improved functional performance, increased lean muscle mass (tone) & ideal body-fat percentage – effectively an optimal state of being.

From my experience there are seven main movements that will help tone, reshape & strengthen your body—*fast*. These movements are the shortest route to total control of your body shape.

They should create the bulk of your training programs as a beginner, or even as a regular lifter.

Combinations of these movements & variations of them can be applied to provide a never-ending selection of exercises to positively overload your muscles to bring about increased strength & improve your performance.

Note:
Always consult a health professional to tailor your training program. In the long run, you will reach your goals faster, saving you time & reducing your chance of injury or illness.

Bang-for-Your-Buck Movements for More Muscle & Fat Loss

Movement 1: Squats

This is arguably the king of movements.

This is the bread & butter of any weight-training program with a focus on body shaping.

It will not only gift you with greater strength & shape, but the by-product of doing a squat effectively, is that your entire body gets a workout.

This is a whole-body exercise with a lower-body focus.

Doing Squats

Definition: A squat is a full-body exercise that focuses on your thigh, hip & buttock muscles—your quads & hamstrings.

Importance: It helps you develop lower-body & core strength, which is essential to numerous bodily processes, everyday life movements & overall health.

Everyday movement: Standing from a chair or the couch. Getting up & down off the toilet. Picking something up from the floor.

Spine protection: When done properly, your back strength will increase, protecting your spine. You strengthen a lifting pattern that benefits your everyday life.

Number of muscle groups used: four main muscle groups & nearly every other muscle in your body - when done properly.

Benefits: You'll build muscle throughout your whole body, burn more fat, maintain mobility & balance, prevent injuries, jump higher, run faster, increase your lower-body strength—the list is virtually endless.

Routine: For best results, split throughout your week while following a structured muscle development program. There are hundreds of ways to apply a squat workout to your routine; foot position, weight/intensity, reps, sets, timing of movement, body angle, rest periods etc. A qualified professional will help you set this up.

Why? You'll achieve a desirable body shape, remain strong in your lower body & through your trunk, perform everyday tasks with ease & improve your sporting performance. Also, the more muscle you have, the more carbs you will be able to eat without getting fat.

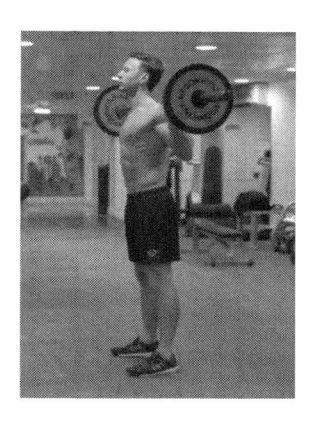 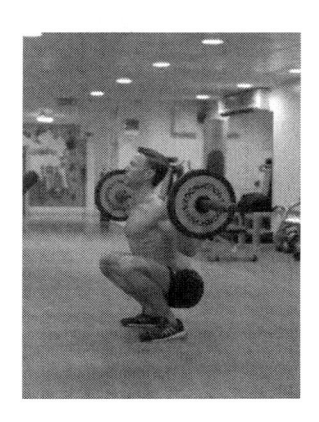

Movement 2: Deadlifts

The dead lift is another mainstay of any quality workout program. One could also argue that this is the king of movements.

Doing Deadlifts

Definition: A weight-training exercise where you lift a weight off the ground from a stable, bent-over position. You lift the weight from a bent over position into a standing position.

Importance: Deadlifts work your arms, legs, butt, abs, shoulders, back, forearms & grip —another complete all-rounder.

Everyday movement: Lifting anything heavy off the floor. Bending over to pick up your briefcase, bag, or backpack. Picking something up from the floor.

Spine protection: Deadlifts improve muscles in your core & back. Strengthening these will prevent injury. With this movement, you should experience massive activation of your back muscles, particularly in your lower back.

Number of muscle groups used: This is a whole body movement, four main muscles groups will get the bulk of the load, in combination with a large number of secondary & stabiliser muscles also being worked.

Benefits: This is the best exercise for working your posterior muscles – the muscles of your back that keep you standing upright. When these are built up over time, they reduce injury potential, support sporting activities by improving explosive strength potential & build serious muscle mass. Deadlifts also improve your body composition, calorie-burn potential, muscle tone, lower-body & core strength & reduce risk of lower-back injury. Again, the list is extensive.

Routine: For best results, split sessions through your week while following a structured muscle-development program. As with the squat there are many ways to apply the deadlift into your routine. Seek the advise of an expert to learn perfect technique, it will benefit you in the long-run.

Why? If you want a healthy, strong back, this exercise should be incorporated into your routine. The great thing about it is that it works your whole body. Your grip & forearms will improve & increase in strength, your posture will be better & even your energy levels will improve. You'll stand more upright, feel stronger & look more confident.

Warning: *If you have ever suffered a back injury or severe back pain, then consult your doctor & a fitness professional before commencing with this movement. As it loads the lower back it is critical that your technique & selection of the variables of this movement are accurate to keep risk of injury to a minimum.*

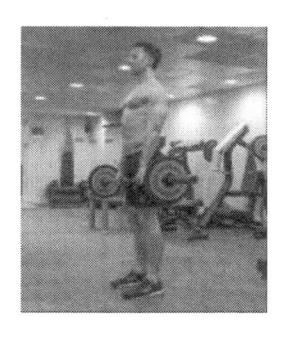 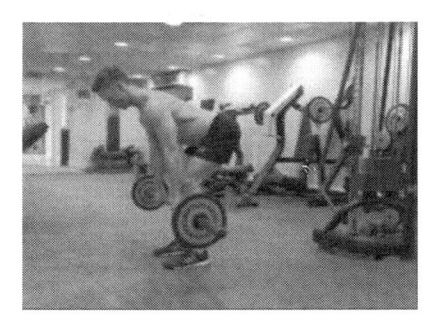

Movement 3: Dips

Dips are an essential part of any well-balanced weight-training program to build a strong upper torso.

Doing Dips

Definition: A dip is a strength-training exercise that focuses on your triceps (back of your arms), chest & front of your shoulders. The name gives you a clue of the movement; you dip your body below the fixed point of your hands & then push yourself up again.

Importance: Dips are important because they contribute to your ability to grow muscle tone in the mentioned areas, which improves strength & power. You hit more than one muscle group, increase your upper-body strength & improve your upper-body shape.

Everyday movement: The ability to hold your own body weight through your arms. Standing up from a low-seated position while using your arms to help. Catching yourself if you slip or fall where all your weight can be loaded through your upper body as you catch yourself (not that this happens to you regularly I hope!)

Spine protection: Dips contribute to core & upper-body strength, so in that respect they could help with some stabilisation of your trunk but the movement focuses mainly on the muscles of the chest & back of your arms.

Number of muscle groups used: At least three main muscle groups—again with added stabiliser & secondary muscle activation, dependent on angle or direction of movement & chosen intensity.

Benefits: Improves overall arm strength & helps improve definition in your chest area. Varying your weight with a weight belt or assisted dip machine or bands will increase muscle mass &/or strength endurance. This will help with body composition, calorie-burn potential & upper-body strength.

Routine: For best results, split routine through your week & follow a structured muscle-development program. Seek the help of a professional to get this set up.

Why? Upper-body strength can diminish rapidly when not challenged. This exercise maintains your upper-body strength while offering the benefit of increased calorie burn, helping you remain or reach the shape you desire. Increasing your ability in this movement will have many positive effects throughout your sporting performance while at the same time making everyday life movements easier.

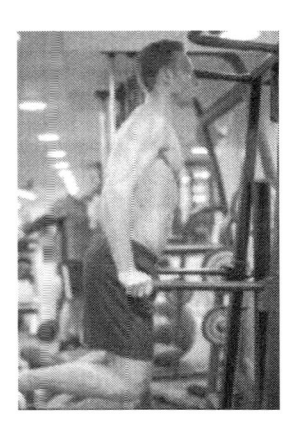 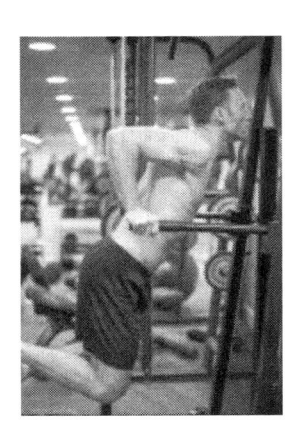

Movements 4: Chin-Ups

Strong back muscles mean more support for your spine. If you want that V-shape physique, then pull-ups & chin-ups are your best friends.

Generally speaking, chin-ups are performed with a supine grip (palms facing up), just inside shoulder-width. Pull-ups are performed with a prone grip (palms facing down), also shoulder-width apart.

Varying the width of your grip brings variation to the exercise & recruitment of muscle fibres.

Chin-ups are smoother on your shoulder joints & stimulate more activation of your biceps. They are easier than pull-ups partly due to the mechanical advantage from hand position, alignment of your shoulders, grip strength & ability to recruit your biceps (front of your arm) more. This is why I suggest starting with chin-ups rather than pull-ups.

Strengthen your chin-ups & then move onto developing your pull-ups. You'll achieve better gains, your shoulders will be happier & you won't be so frustrated by the slowness of the progress from pull-ups.

Doing Chin-Ups

Definition: These focus on the upper body. You perform them using a pull-up bar by pulling yourself up from a straightened-arm (hanging) position, bringing your chest to the bar, by fully bending at your elbows (flexion)

Importance: Chin-ups improve upper-body & core strength, power & force in your back & arm muscles. They're important for postural alignment & also improve grip strength & forearm development.

Everyday movement: Pulling yourself up from a seated position; any pulling activity where you move a weight toward your body, for example, moving furniture, pulling yourself over obstacles, or tug-of-war…if you like that kind of thing.

Spine protection: These provide a massive overload for your back muscles, so they help stabilise your spine & improve posture.

Number of muscle groups used: Three main muscle groups—back, biceps (front of upper arms) & shoulders. Your trunk muscles will also get a workout. When you really get going, your hamstrings will also try to help out.

Benefits: Upper-body strength increases. You'll notice improvement in the muscle tone & shape of your upper body particularly your back. This movement will elevate your metabolic rate & calorie burn plus help towards maintaining good posture & a healthy spine.

Routine: For best results, use a split routine spread throughout your week. Seek the help of a professional to help set this up effectively. As an absolute minimum you should be able to complete 1 full range pull-up of your own body-weight. If you cant then its time to get training!

Why? Any pulling movement you perform in everyday life will be improved—opening doors, pulling on your pants & moving furniture will all become an extremely easy part of everyday life – if they are not already?

(A side thought… On top of the above mentioned benefits, if you ever happen to be hanging off a cliff at any point in your life you will at that point be very glad you had practiced this exercise as you would be able to pull yourself up & save your own life!)

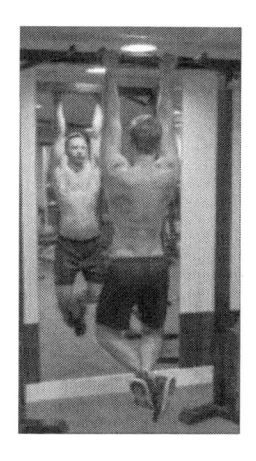 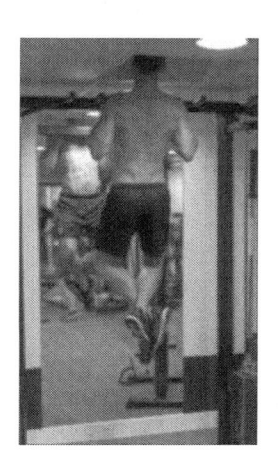

Movement 5: Rows

This is a weight-training exercise that helps your body become the strong, lean force you have always wanted it to be. It is a great exercise to not only increase muscle tone in your back & arms but to also support optimal posture.

Doing Rows

Definition: A bent-over row is a weight-training exercise that works on your back muscle groups & also strengthens your core, biceps, grip & forearms.

Importance: Rows will strengthen your back & grip, which in turn improves your dead lift & helps you build more muscle in all the right places for correct postural alignment. It teaches you to stabilise your spine while you're in a forward-bend position (e.g., picking up a briefcase, suitcase, or shopping bags) without risk to your back.

Everyday movement: Mimics the act of lifting something heavy from the ground & pulling something close to the trunk of your body.

Spine protection: Targets the muscle groups in the back for lifting & remaining upright. Strengthens the muscles running up your spine & increases tone in your postural muscles, making you stand more upright…& look taller.

Muscle groups used: Upper & middle back, depending on the focus & angle of the movement, as well as arm muscles, shoulders, grip & forearm.

Benefits: Rows help turn your back into a strong center for your body, prevent injury to your spine, increase arm strength, improve muscle tone in your back & arms, maintain & increase grip strength. They also improve body composition & increase calorie-burn potential through the added muscle stimulation & growth. As the back is a large muscle (group) the more tone you achieve within these muscles the more calories & fat you will burn throughout your day.

Routine: For best results, integrate this movement into a structured weight-training plan. For best results have a qualified professional periodise your training sessions for you.

Why? This is a movement that you will perform every day of your life—unless your lower back is already compromised. Performing this movement in a controlled, progressive way will help you recover from back injury or decrease your chances of suffering from back pain. It will help you maintain good posture & make it easier for you to reach & maintain optimal body-fat stores.

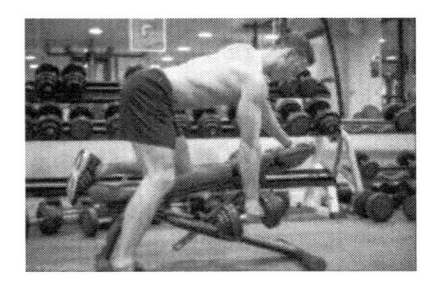 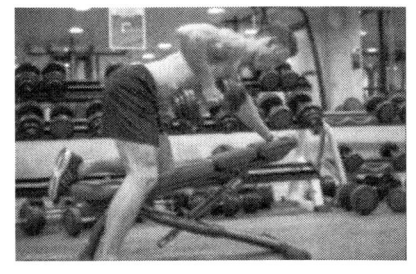

Movements 6: Bench Press

Doing Bench Press

Definition: A bench press is an upper-body exercise where you lie on your back & push/resist weights, the main focus of the movement is on your chest.

Importance: This exercise improves your strength through the pushing motion. It is probably the most popular upper-body exercise. This is the body-shaping exercise of choice for most men as it stimulates growth in the chest muscles bringing about a vision & feeling of a much larger upper body. Every athletic man wants a big bench weight & a big chest.

For women this is less of a concern but it could be argued that toning the muscles in this area will help to keep the breast area more pert. In general women tend to focus more on toning their legs & keeping their butt shapely.

Both men & women should be strong in this movement to ensure optimal muscular & structural integrity.

Everyday movement: Lifting your own body weight from the floor when you are face down—a push up. Being able to push up from the floor with stability & strength or effectively resist an object or person that is coming toward you, or to even repel them away from you.

Spine protection: This exercise provides less focus on training the muscles surrounding the spine than the previous movements. The bench press strengthens shoulders, arms & chest—all of which are fundamental to core power. If overdone, as commonly happens with those who want bigger chest muscles, it can be counterproductive to posture & your spine. It is important that your training is balanced between pushing & pulling movements to build your body shape evenly & ensure a healthy spine. If this is not managed effectively, you'll experience bad posture, back pain & long layoffs from the gym or your sport, which will likely result in increased body fat.

Muscle groups used: Bench pressing works your pectorals (chest muscles), triceps (back of arm) & anterior deltoids (front of shoulders).

Benefits: Bench pressing builds strength in your arms & chest. It improves power, bone density in your upper body & athletic performance. It can also support ideal body shape, calorie burn & fat loss.

Routine: Split throughout your week while following a structured muscle-development program. As mentioned, this is a great exercise but should not be overdone. Balance your pushing routines with pulls to ensure long-term back health, good posture & improved sporting performance through correct structural alignment. A good strength coach will be able to help you with this. Variation of this exercise will bring continued progression & improved structural balance to your upper body musculature.

Why? *'If you don't use it, you lose it'* – is an old saying that rings true. Upper-body strength diminishes over time if you don't keep challenging it. This movement effectively works several upper-body muscles, providing an effective way to shape your upper body & keep it strong.

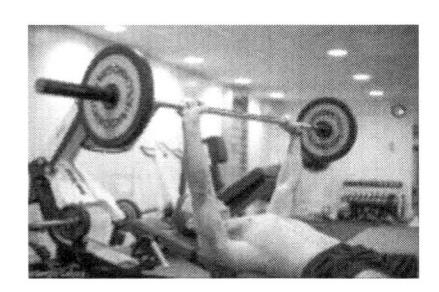 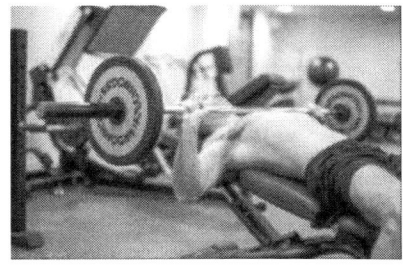

Movement 7: Abdominals

The final movement works the abs, or abdominal muscles. These are the ones people often struggle with the most. Not to fear, when combined with the other exercises I have suggested above & the rest of the information within this book you'll experience a rapid improvement in the way your stomach area looks if you happen to be carrying a little extra around the middle right now.

Definition: Your abs are the muscles between your chest & your pelvis. Exercises that focus on this area are usually completed purely for aesthetic reasons, however there is a smarter way to train where you not only have great looking abs but also functional strength throughout your trunk muscles that improve your physical performance, & reduce potential back injury. Combining the techniques & theories I provide you within this book & training your abdominals effectively will result in visible muscle definition in your abdominal region.

Importance: Ab movements should help strengthen your core & support your spine. They work in coordination with your back muscles to stabilise your trunk area & therefore take stress off the vertebrae & discs of your spine. Optimal abdominal muscle function should also support your internal organs & protect them from injury from sudden intense movement or sporting situations.

Everyday movement: Bending, twisting, lifting your body off the floor when face up or getting out of bed when face up, sitting upright. Your abdominals *should* be working intermittently all day long, as they should stabilise your spine before any movement occurs. Your deep abdominal muscles (TVA) should contract 0.01 seconds before any movement from your limbs.

Spine protection: Effective abdominals support your spine. Effectively trained stronger abs mean a reduction in back injuries when you play sports or participate in other physical activities. It is *uncommon* for a sports professional or everyday person to incur a 'trunk' injury, but it is very *common* for either community to suffer a back injury. Strengthening the entire abdominal wall rather than just the rectus abdominus (muscle that makes the 6 pack visible) will lessen the chances of back injury & actually provide a better foundation for longer more sustained progression within all exercise & physical performance.

Muscle groups used: I segment the abdominal region into upper area, oblique's, lower area & transverse abdominus. However, they are one unit of muscles that work in combination with each other & surrounding muscles. There are also deep abdominal muscles, as explained earlier. For optimal health & physical performance you would be wise to periodise your training to achieve balance across all muscle groups throughout your trunk.

Although your abdominal wall is connected—your upper & lower abs are not separate, they are one muscle—I refer to them in areas in order to focus exercises & strengthen specific areas of your abdominal wall. After isolating an area in order to increase strength you should always integrate that strength into a whole body movement, in the process you strengthen your entire system.

Benefits: Abdominal conditioning is one of the best ways to strengthen your core muscles in isolation. Bear in mind that you must also integrate the strength of these muscles into your everyday movements. I go over this in more detail in my training programs. If you want to reduce aches, pains & back injury, then specific abdominal conditioning is essential.

Routine: Perform abdominal exercises daily or split throughout your week if you are following a structured muscle-development program. Provided you have optimal function & strength in your abdominal wall, a good strength coach will be able to integrate abdominal conditioning into the main lifts of your workout.

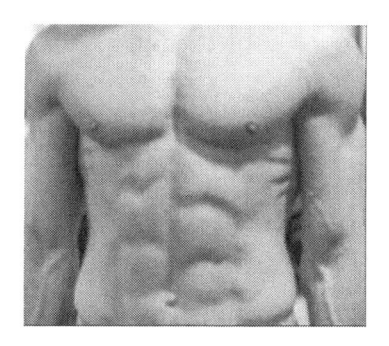

Why? The main reason for abdominal exercises is to ensure they are strong enough to stabilise your spine as you perform high-intensity lifts or movements, such as a heavy squatting or playing your chosen sport.

Other reasons are for better body composition, calorie-burn potential & aesthetics—because lets be honest, most people would to have a six-pack.

Connected

Your abdominal wall is connected, not defined into sections. People often talk about their upper abs, lower abs, oblique's & deep abdominal muscles. All these areas are actually connected & function simultaneously in movement patterns.

The only reason to segment them is so that you can feel where certain exercises hit you & also focus on increasing strength in specific areas, in order to improve sporting performance, increase structural integrity of your spine or support/rehabilitate a back injury.

Heavy-load, low-rep training, for example, stimulate the body to grow muscle, strength & power. Depending on the tempo of the movement this type of training stimulates fast twitch muscles fibers. These fibers are more receptive to weight training & will respond more quickly to training stimulus.

While your body is being worked in this way the muscles of your trunk should contract quickly just before the movement is initiated to support your spine.

If your abs don't perform optimally then you are at high risk for spinal injury. Your spine is left bare & exposed. This can be eradicated by good strength training within a well-structured training program.

Warning: Back Injury-Prevention Techniques

It makes sense that the stronger your abs are, the better they'll perform—& the less likely that you'll sustain a serious spinal injury—&, in turn, the better you'll perform.

It's important that you work all areas of your abdominal wall so they are in proportional strength to one another.

This strength also needs to be matched by lower-back strength. If you do not manage this, you're setting yourself up for an injury.

There are lots of specific abdominal exercises that you can perform, but there are only two questions that determine your selection of exercise.

    i. What movement is going to improve the stability
       of my back or support my athletic performance?
       – Function.
    ii. What movement is going to create a better-looking
       six-pack? – Aesthetics.

Each exercise recruits specific portions of your abdominal wall. Although your abdominals are interconnected & should function as one unit or team, you can focus movements into targeted areas in order to strengthen that area & therefore strengthen the movement pattern that area is involved in, or simply improve the look of that area.

I use six main movements to work the abdominal region of the body. When performed properly & within a balanced exercise program these exercises will strengthen your core & effectively support your spine:

A little warning: With lower back injuries you would likely not strengthen your abdominals in the way I describe below. You would use plank or lengthening exercises that strengthen your abs in a lengthened neutral spine position.

This is why yoga can be good for low back pain as it teaches you to be strong but in a lengthened & sometimes stretched position.

So bearing in mind you do not have back pain or issues of any kind here is a list of effective abdominal building exercises:

1. Crunch: Best performed over a stability ball or BOSU. WARNING: If you have ever suffered a low back injury you may need to avoid this exercise for a period of time. With correct rehabilitation you will be able to use this movement again but not until you have healed your back issue & balanced your core strength of lower back & abdominal muscles.
2. Side bends (side flexion): Standing or kneeling using dumbbells or cables.
3. Rotation: A wood-chop motion with upper body, lateral leg drops with lower body. Using cables, dumbbells or medicine balls.
4. Reverse curls: Leg raises, knee tucks using cables or medicine balls.
5. Static strength: Variations of plank / holding static positions.
6. Deep abdominal training: TVA (Transverse Abdominis)—you'd be wise to incorporate your pelvic floor muscle here as well - Principle 9.

In regard to effective abdominal condition your main aim should be functional capability & strength. Only then should you have any concern for aesthetics. If your abdominals function optimally then your back will be safer for it. Once your abdominals are performing as they should, you will have more freedom to train harder.

Your first job is to understand & determine how well your abdominals work for you. If you or your health professional highlight a weakness within your abdominal wall then you will need to isolate, strengthening that weakness, & then integrate, use that added strength within a main movement pattern, for instance a squat, deadlift or lunge.

Other areas of your body will appear stronger when your core strength is at optimum.

Your body works synergistically—you could even argue that no muscle ever works alone. Your core musculature is at the foundation of all your movements.

If the foundations are not strong then the entire building is weak. Even if you have a strong chest or back, but your core musculature is not adequate, you will not be able to tap into that strong chest or back effectively.

Its like a building that has the worlds strongest steel for its walls & structure but the foundation is weak – the smallest of earthquakes could crumble the building or at least damage the integrity of the building. It will then no longer function as well.

Stabilise...

Stabiliser muscles contract to provide support so active muscles can do their jobs effectively. Abs are the supporting muscles of your body; they are involved in nearly every movement you perform. Your deep abdominal muscles should contract right before any movement of your arm(s) or leg(s).

Remember, the chain will always break at the weakest link. Or another way to put it is; You are only as strong as your weakest link.

If your abs are the weakest link, then your entire body is weak. Everything is interrelated & connected through your trunk.

Increase the effectiveness of your abdominals & all other exercise techniques will become easier, essentially your results will increase. The body must progress as a whole, or it will simply break down with injury or illness. In fact this is a problem for a lot of people.

It is common to have a favorite body part to work, or a favorite exercise. But what this usual equates to is over exercise of that area of exercise. Other areas are left to atrophy or are not of equal strength.

The body will only allow for a certain amount of asymmetry. Once you apply balance to your training programs, movements & muscles you can then achieve an even growth. If balanced, your body & brain will allow growth to continue without asymmetry being the limiting factor.

The stronger your trunk (core muscles) the stronger your body as a whole.

Muscle mass is one of the most important factors in determining longevity. As a statistic, lean muscle mass is more important than cholesterol, heart disease or even your blood pressure.[1,2,3]

---

1 http://www.ncbi.nlm.nih.gov/pubmed/22030953

2 http://www.ncbi.nlm.nih.gov/pubmed/24997614

3 http://www.ncbi.nlm.nih.gov/pubmed/24707476

Well-Oiled Machine...

The more muscle you have, the more your body works like a well-oiled machine. On top of that, your muscle mass helps keep many other important elements, like your diet, in check.

If you keep your diet exactly the same as it is now & add in an effective weight-training program, you'll still notice a radical improvement in your body shape.

Improve your diet along with the training & you compound your results, giving yourself even greater success.

I always explain to my clients that the more muscle they have the more calories they will burn everyday, the more protected their joints & the better they will be able to perform.

Principle Exercise 13
Exercise Choice & Variables

If you want optimal results in the quickest possible time it is critically important that you vary your training stimulus.

A training program or an individual exercise is only good for the time it takes for your body to adapt to it.

This means that there is an optimal curve of improvement for each exercise, movement & training program.

Once the peak has been reached from that stimulus it is time to alter the variable(s).

You could alter the variables of the movement, for example the speed at which you are performing the movement, or the rest period between sets, or the sequence of exercises you have lined up etc.

Point being that in order to keep improving you must vary how your body (& brain) challenged.

The rate at which you should vary stimulus depends heavily on the individual. This is where working with a skilled training coach is invaluable. They will be able to periodise your training program (have a long-term plan) to ensure continued success.

A general rule of thumb is that most people adapt to a training program in approximately six workouts. This means that you can set the program & diligently follow it for six workouts, you must then alter stimulus in order to keep getting optimal gains.

The intricate details around planning & variation of training programs is vast. There are many books written solely about each of these two topics.

For now your approach should be to apply a specific routine, which you follow for a maximum of six workouts.

At that point set up a new routine. Practice this long-term & you will consistently stimulate success from your training programs.

Principle 13
I Consistently Vary My Training Stimulus

The key to long-term success with your health & fitness is meticulous
planning & consistent variation.

The truth is that each individual requires unique alterations to each lifestyle tip, exercise plan, nutrition & supplement plan.

A book like this one can provide an essential starting point of knowledge. However to constantly make progress within any endeavor a requirement of consistent learning is mandatory.

You must consistently vary your training stimulus by sourcing a coach or number of coaches who are experts. They will guide you by providing continuous snippets of information that you can easily apply to your life.

Begin to live by this principle by applying the information I have provided so far.

If you decide to follow my blog, receive my emails, connect with me through social media then I will continue to enable your progress toward living at optimal health & fitness.

You are probably already aware that a coach will get you to your goal quicker than you could by going it alone.

In order to live by this principle of 'Consistently Varying Your Training Stimulus' you will need outside help. The learning curve around health & fitness is endless. No-one person can know everything there is to know & the information is constantly advancing.

Be wise & align yourself with the best teachers available to you. That way the information you will receive will always aid you & you will have a consistent selection of variables when designing your training programs.

Chapter 8:
The Theory behind Exercise

Training gives us an outlet for suppressed energies created by stress, and thus tones the spirit, just as exercise conditions the body.

—*Arnold Schwarzenegger*

Exercise is easy, right? All you have to do is run for a while, work out on machines, or lift a few weights a couple of times a week.

This approach may work for a little while but what you will find is that more structure & a planned approach will bring you continued results long-term.

It takes many years of diligent practice, if not a lifetime, to come to some level of mastery within any discipline. The same principle applies in regards to program design.

There is not one way that suits all & answers all questions. The program that you start today is only good for as long as it takes you to adapt to it.

What I mean by this is that you must change your training regime regularly. The movements, the sets, the reps, the rest periods, the recovery time, the intensity etc. Only through continuous intelligent well-timed change can you keep making progress. Apply Principle 13 throughout your training program plan.

You have to understand the biomechanics of exercise in order to streamline your efforts, so that you can get the most "burn for your buck" while building lots of lean muscle.

Obviously consulting an expert in this field is the quickest way to learn methods that work & get the results you desire in the shortest possible time. However, it is always helpful to have an understanding of some basic principles.

I provide you with the baseline methods to consider when planning your training program.

Remember, your design depends on your goal & that there are many ways to reach it.

To get you going, consider the following variables when taking on a new training regime.

Working with Sets & Reps

A *set* is one variable used by fitness professionals to describe the number of times you perform an exercise within a workout.

This means how many times you repeat an exercise. You could perform many sets of each exercise in one workout.

A *rep*, short for *repetition*, is another term used to describe a workout's structure & organisation. It describes how many times you will perform a certain movement within each set.

If your plan is to do ten squats three times, you would be doing three sets of ten reps.

Here's how you need to treat sets & reps when you work out.

- Using sets & reps, you'll be able to scale your workout according to your current ability, goals & fitness/health threshold.

- When you plan your sets & reps properly, you achieve a more efficient response from your training. This will effectively appear like you have sped up your results.

- Focus on performing perfect reps & in turn perfect sets so that you build useful muscle. Essentially you'll be strong in perfect postural alignment. This is ideal to keep your risk of injury as low as possible.

- The five main features to focus on when designing a training program: the number of sets per body part, the number of reps per completed set, rest periods, tempo (the speed at which you perform each rep) & frequency of training.

- Sets & reps have an inverse relationship. The higher the reps the lower the number of sets you perform, i.e. 4 sets of 12. Or vice versa, the lower the reps the higher the number of sets you perform, i.e. 10 sets of 3.

Setting the Sets

General Rule for Sets & Reps

You could apply an endless combination of sets & rep schemes. Many books have been written about these two topics alone.

A general starting place is to aim for eight to twelve reps per set & three sets per exercise. For starters you could complete four to six exercises per workout.

Remember that this is a general explanation to help get you started. The best thing you can do is to hire a professional to set up a structured training program for you. That way, you know you're performing the correct number of movements with the correct form & at the right speed in order to obtain results as quickly as possible.

Start with the guidelines provided above, & as your experience increases so can the complexity of your sets-&-reps structure.

Every exercise program must be specific to the individual for maximum return on time invested.

Continuous Progression

One way to stimulate steady progression is to attempt to perform one more repetition each time you do a set.

Keep in mind that you don't lose quality at the expense of quantity. This means that you must perform every rep with good form. Always aim to apply perfect technique.

Perfect Practice Makes Perfect

When you increase your reps by one at every workout, you're increasing volume of work on the muscles involved. If you can increase by more than one rep & still keep your form, then do so.

The more reps you manage, the more muscle you'll pack on. Whenever you apply more volume to a working muscle it will grow. As you perform more reps, you'll need to adjust the weight to continue to work in your desired rep range.

For instance if you squat 30kg for 10 reps first attempt, your next workout you'll be aiming to complete 11 reps & so on.

Once you've reached the top of your rep range, which is twelve sticking with my earlier example, you'll need to increase the weight in order to still get a challenge from within the desired rep range (eight to twelve).

The rep range determines the physiological response from your body. At the same time the body shape you're attempting to achieve will determine what rep range & style of training you perform. See the connection.

For more structured & tailored training programs, you'd save yourself the most time & effort by hiring the best professional you can get your hands on.

Rest for Better Progressions

In terms of exercising for body composition or health & fitness benefits, a logical thought would be to start exercising & train as hard & long as you can. However if you want long-term success a smarter approach is required.

To set the scene imagine two different resistance training approaches:

1. Lifting a heavy weight that you can only lift 4 or 5 times (4 or 5 rep max)
2. Lifting a lighter weight that you can lift 10 or more times.

The first approach requires much more neural drive – the medical specialty of neurology focuses on the nervous system & that is what I am talking about here. Lifting a weight that you can only perform less than six reps with will require much more of your nervous system (more neural drive is required to power that movement) than a weight that you can lift 10 or more times.

With this type of training you will stimulate more of a neurological response. You will strengthen your system & the power that can be directed to your muscles. You will get stronger.

A general rule of thumb is that if you are training heavy–for instance, with a one- to five-rep max– then you will require more recovery time between sets.

It takes your nervous system approximately five times longer to recover than your muscular system.

When you lift heavy as explained above, you are mostly training neural drive. You are conditioning your nervous system to generate more output. At the same time you will also be working your fast twitch muscle fibers, which are more responsive to training stimulus than your slow twitch muscle fibers.

This is great training if you want to increase your overall strength. Keep in mind that you would only do this for an average of three weeks for women & two weeks for men within a training cycle.

The strain on your system is high & you would not train year round in this way. A good periodisation program would take care of this for you. Periodisation is the long-term planning of a training program. For example, for X amount of weeks you will perform strength building exercises followed by X amount of weeks of training to build muscular endurance, & so on.

When you are training with heavy weights for low repetition sets, you require two- to five-minute rest periods between each set. This allows your body to sufficiently recover for a quality next set.

For rep ranges of eight or more, you require up to two minutes or less rest periods. This is because for the higher rep ranges you are overloading your muscular system & not as much focus is placed on your nervous system, therefore the rest periods can be shorter.

For rep ranges of twenty or more, you require sixty-seconds or less rest periods. This is because the exercise fatigues your muscular endurance system & your muscles need less time to recover than your nervous system does.

Remember these are general guidelines & there is an endless variation structure that you can apply to these variables depending on training goal or sporting event.

Plan your rest periods correctly for optimal return on your training program. Again, a professional will help you set this up properly.

A little trick would be to complete a two-week strength phase followed by three to four weeks of muscular endurance. This will increase the amount of weight you are able to lift in preparation for the endurance phase.

The more weight you lift the more muscle you will build the more calories you will burn the more fat you will burn or effectively never store in the first place.

Remember attempting to increase the weight you lift should not affect your technique. Do not lose quality at the expense of quantity.

The Frequency of Exercise

I am often asked, "How many times per week should I be training to get results?"

The answer lies in your level of experience & type of result(s) you desire. If you are a beginner, then you require less frequent training, about three times per week.

A day's rest between each workout will likely work best for someone who is just starting out.

Once you have been lifting (training) for six months or more—or as soon as your health, fitness & recovery time allows—you can step that up.

A seasoned pro may train as often as three times a day, on three out of every five days.

It takes years to build up your body's tolerance to that level & volume of training. Also, genetics allow some people to grow muscle easily or recover quicker, while others aren't so lucky.

A general rule of thumb is to start at three times per week. Once you feel you can perform another session, add it in. Again, for optimal results in the quickest possible time it is always best to periodise your training program.

One example of periodising your training would be to ramp up your training volume, in terms of how much you do within a workout, how much weight you lift & how frequently you train for a planned period of time.

You would increase volume for a period of time, for instance two to four weeks, depending on your training style. Then you ease off for a week or two, then repeat the cycle.

You wouldn't train three times a day, seven days a week, 365 days a year. Your body would break!

General Rule for Training Frequency:

Studies show that if your workouts last for more than one hour you could be negatively affecting your cortisol curve causing more stress than good & hindering your long-term success.[1, 2, 3]

1 http://www.ncbi.nlm.nih.gov/pubmed/24715614

2 http://www.ncbi.nlm.nih.gov/pubmed/25144130

3 http://www.ncbi.nlm.nih.gov/pubmed/25380472

One study demonstrated that prolonged workloads increase injury rates & incidence of illness.[1]

If your workouts last approximately one hour then the table below will help you determine the frequency of your workouts:

LEVEL	AMOUNT
Beginners **(Under 1 year of experience)**	3 sessions per week, 1 day rest between workouts
Intermediate (1+ year of experience)	4+ workouts per week Resting 2 days out of every six. The training split of rest & workout days can be applied with.
Advanced (2+ years of experience)	8+ sessions per week This can include training more than once per day. For example 8 workouts completed within a 6 day cycle with 2 rest days, you can play with the position of the rest days to best suit your style, recovery time, schedule & goal.

Training eight days straight my not be the wisest decision. Resting optimally will bring you optimal results from the time & effort you invest.

A Little Tip to Maintain Progression

To maintain muscle firmness & at the same time keep the muscle in a prepared state for movement (commonly known in bodybuilding as a pump), don't go longer than two days without working that muscle. Otherwise, you will begin to lose strength & it may start to feel softer & less able.

In fact it has been demonstrated that muscle atrophy (wastage & decline in function) can happen quickly & suddenly, especially when the muscle is not used regularly.[1]

It is even suggested that you can lose up to eighty percent of your strength in as little as two weeks if you are new to regular exercise.[2]

Hit your muscles regularly with pre-defined movements. Even if that involves doing only one set.

I'm not talking about attacking a muscle for growth everyday. What I am suggesting is slightly challenging the muscles on a daily basis while thoroughly thrashing each muscle within a structured planned workout program.

If you are strapped for time, one concentrated set of an exercise can help maintain blood flow to the muscle which is great for healing & peak performance, muscle mass & readiness for activity.

You've probably noticed this in other areas of your life:

'The less you do the less you want to do – The more you do the more you want to do'.

I have found that adding in these little & often routines, between main workouts, has a compounding long-term positive effect.

---

1 http://ajcn.nutrition.org/content/91/4/1123S.full

2 http://www.livestrong.com/article/383660-how-fast-do-you-lose-muscle-by-not-training/

Principle Exercise 14
Mini Routine

Here are a few examples of exercises that you could use on a daily basis to stimulate muscle function & reduce muscle atrophy (wasting or softness).

You do not need equipment, just some floor space & some energy.

Complete at least one set of eight to twenty repetitions of each movement every day.

1. Bodyweight Squat
Squat with your own body weight to work your legs, butt & core muscles—a great all-rounder. Play around with the width of your feet to focus on different areas of your thighs & butt.

You can also adjust the other variables I mentioned earlier like tempo (speed of movement). Try lowering yourself to the floor slowly, 10 seconds, then squatting back to a standing position. Repeat that a few times & feels your quads working.

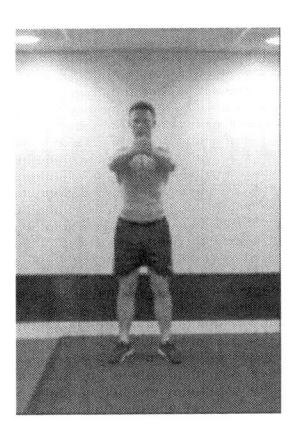 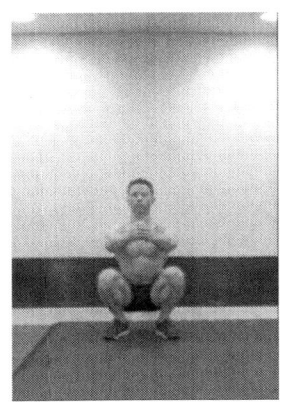

2. Push Up

Press your own body weight away from the floor to improve chest, arm & core strength. Try to keep you deep abdominal muscle activated as you perform the movement, this will strengthen your core muscles & protect your spine.

Again play around with the variables I suggested earlier. For instance, raise your foot position by placing your feet on a step (bottom of a staircase). This will work different fibres in your chest & arms, focusing the movement on the upper area of your chest. You can also adjust the height of that step over time giving you variation & room for continuous progression.

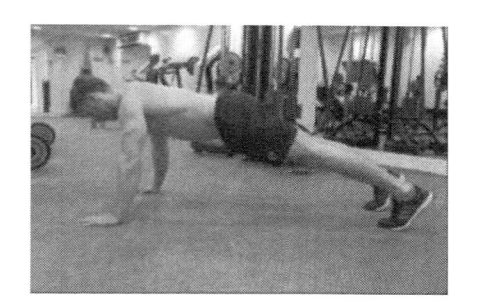 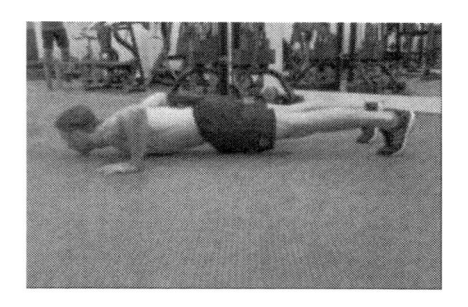

3. Double Crunch

This exercise focuses on your abdominal muscles. The curling up of your upper body works the upper area of your abs while the lifting & tucking of your legs & knees works the lower area.

These movements when combined, fully recruit your rectus abdominus – the abdominal muscle that runs from under your sternum (chest bone) to your pubic bone. This is the muscle associated with the six-pack look.

Stretch out as you reach the extended position (image 1) for every repetition, even slightly arch your back when your legs & head are in contact with the floor.

This will work the full range of motion of this muscle. This is important, as excessive crunch type exercises will shorten this muscle pulling your spine into flexion – bad posture.

Fully lengthening for every rep encourages the muscle to remain at full length while at the same time strengthening it. You will also achieve more aesthetic development when you work the full range of movement.

NOTE: If you suffer with lower back pain this exercise is not advised as it places the lower spine into flexion, which could worsen your condition. Seek the advice of a professional when suffering with back pain.

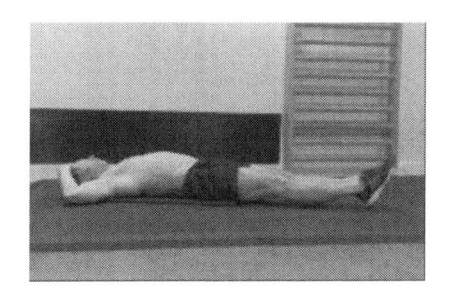 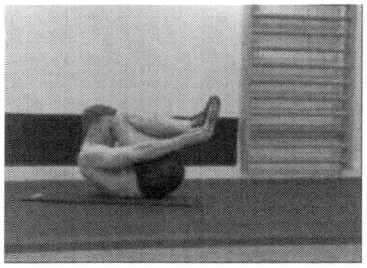

4. Prone Cobra or Sky Diver

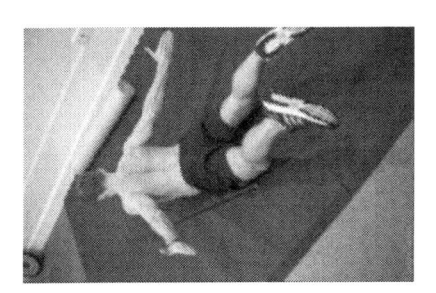

This exercise will work your back muscles & if performed regularly will improve your posture.

You can perform reps of the movement, lifting your yourself from the floor into the extended position (Image 1) & then lowering yourself back down.

Or longer holds of one or more minutes for this movement, where you hold the position demonstrated in the image —again, vary what you do over time in order to keep progressing.

Principle 14
I Enjoy Daily Exercise

Variances in the speed at which you perform a movement, the number of repetitions, the sets you perform, the length of the rest periods between sets & the angle at which you perform the movement will affect the muscles involved - how they develop, how they perform & how they look.

For example, lets use a push-up. You can perform a push up from your knees, or bring your knees closer to your hands, or perform the movement from your feet, or have your feet raised. Each position will challenge your body in a different way.

Find your challenge position, the closer your knees are to your hands the easier the movement, & then determine how many reps you can perform in that shape.

Altering the position will determine how many reps you can complete. Aim to complete more reps over time. Alter the position & alter the reps.

Varying the rep range stimulates your muscles in a different way, resulting in a different look, feel & function to your physique.

Feel free to play around with these factors on a daily basis or within a structured plan. The main point being that you are improving.

Complete these movements daily to build strength & help shape your "Greek-god body"

The Optimal Principle here is to stimulate your body daily through exercise. Even if it only lasts a few minutes make sure you exercise daily. This could be a long walk in a calming environment like the local woods, fields or park.

Solution 3: Nutrition

Chapter 9:
Nutrition or Bust

The food you eat can be either the safest and most powerful form of medicine or the slowest form of poison.

—Ann Wigmore

Now that you have a greater understanding of your exercise routines, it's the perfect time to move on to section three of the Optimalism Principles.

In this section, we'll take a hard look at nutrition & the role it plays in your life. You may not know it yet, but the saying, "You are what you eat," is scary in its accuracy.

Look at Obesity

The Western world is fat—too fat—& getting fatter by the year. According to the Health & Social Care Information Centre, obesity has reached epidemic proportions in the UK. Now, some 24 percent of men & 26 percent of women are considered obese.

Obesity can be defined as a medical condition in which excess body fat has accumulated to the point that it causes harmful side effects.

These effects can be anything from high blood pressure (hypertension), breathing difficulties, to heart disease, cancer, diabetes & metabolic dysfunction.

Why is the obesity epidemic running rampant in our towns & cities?

- Modern grocery stores supply easy access to cheap, high-energy foods that are aggressively marketed to a "busy" public. It's easier to microwave a meal than to consider an hour of cooking time.

- Modern jobs are arguably way more stressful than in previous generations. It's estimated that we endure one hundred times more stress than our grandparents.

- Many careers require near-constant sitting, so inactivity has become a part of life.

- Through technology, we have automated movement. We get in a car/bus/subway/train that carries us to work, escalators that lift us up stairs & even moving sidewalks to do the walking for us. No wonder we're getting fatter—we've cut out so many forms of natural movement out of our daily lives.

   ...Will we all look like the humans in the movie **Wall**-E *in twenty years' time?*

Recognise the Signs?

You need to overcome three main causes of obesity if you're going to drop your excess body fat; build quality, lean muscle; & shape your physically fit appearance.

The first two are toxicity & stress—the enemies of any healthy individual even before overeating & obesity take effect.

Let's take a closer look:

- Toxicity levels are rampant. Toxins surround you.

The moment toxins enter your body, they can begin to cause harm. Depending on the toxin, it can even burn you on the way in.

For the most part, they roam around your arteries & find an internal organ to damage.

To prevent this, your body collects & excretes toxins as quickly as possible. When you aren't living a healthy lifestyle, your body's natural ability to perform this task is inhibited.

This means that your body doesn't collect & excrete toxins as it should. To ensure this vital process happens optimally, it's your job as guardian of your body to make sure that you have adequate vitamin & mineral levels.

Amino acids are a massive part of this detoxification process.

You get amino acids from protein (predominantly meat & fish) & you can also supplement them.

Most people are deficient in at least one vitamin or mineral, alongside amino acid deficiency.

Where should all this come from?

It should come from your diet. However, for the modern person who lives in a big city, two main factors prevent this from being the case.

1) Bad Food Choices Lead to Bad Choices

When you don't feel your best, you often turn to something you know you shouldn't be eating—like chocolate or crisps/potato chips.

You'll usually do this for the instant sugar, salt or fat rush in your blood stream that signals to your brain that you can relax, or that you are being rewarded for something good.

Basically, these foods make us *think* we feel good, which then makes us *feel* like all is well.

On top of that, marketing is so aggressive that it has to have an affect on our choices.

Less-than-ideal foods are made to look so appetising, tasty & affordable—& in some cases, even good for you.

The lower your personal level of health, the more likely you are to make bad choices & bad choices in general. This relates to food, work & your private life.

The opposite is also true. The healthier you are, the better choices you make all around & your life takes an upward turn.

One example I can use to explain my point here is the expression 'gut feeling'. You will know what I'm talking about if you've ever been faced with a decision & it just didn't feel like the right thing to do – in your gut.

What's going on here?

As around 90 percent of your neurotransmitters are made in your gut this clearly demonstrates the link between your brain (decision making) & your gut (digestion).

Your neurotransmitters are chemicals that basically transmit signals from within your body. They determine your mood & how well you're able to concentrate & focus. The better your neurotransmitters are performing the better you will perform, physically – mentally – emotionally.[1]

---

1 http://www.scientificamerican.com/article/gut-second-brain/

The more health promoting your diet the healthier your gut will be. The healthier your gut the more optimal your neurotransmitter production will be.

Improve the health of your gut & you will improve the function of your mind.

On top of this around 75 percent of your nervous system is located within your gut. So not only will you improve your memory, ability to focus & productivity but you will also get sick less & have fewer days off work & training due to illness.

Top Tip:
Follow the dietary advice of people who pass all three criteria below:

   i. Look like they know what they're talking about.
  ii. Have results with others that prove they know what they're talking about.
 iii. Make logical sense when they explain their theories to you—you understand everything. They are able to teach *you* what *they* know.

Start making better food choices today, keep making them day after day & reap the rewards in the weeks, months & years to come.

Start taking care of your gut, which in turn takes care of your brain today.

2) The Quality of the Food.

So even if you start making better food choices, sometimes there's another roadblock to overcome.

Low-nutrient food (even if your choice was the real healthy option) day after day takes its toll on your body in that you don't have what you need in order to reach optimal state.

So what I mean here is that you may choose a chicken breast or a processed food, but if you choose the cheapest chicken breast or cheapest meal you can get your hands on it may be filled with chemicals & a concoction of poisonous *health damaging* substances which do you harm.

I call this 'Dealth'. Death in stealth mode! This is when you are being dealt a slow death in a very subtle way through processed chemical foods.

This process will slowly but surely bring about ill health & complication into your life.

Foods that use more energy & digestive enzymes to digest them than they provide have been referred to as "displacement foods." Weston A. Price offers plenty of evidence about these foods in his book Nutrition and Physical Degeneration.

Price demonstrated, through extensive research with primitive tribes who come into contact with modern civilisation, how inadequate nutrition causes facial deformities & underdevelopment of body & brain tissue.

Price was an orthodontist—a specialised dentist focusing on bite & jaw alignment. What he found as he traveled the world is that when a diet is altered to lower-nutrient, high-energy, sugary foods, the human body fails to grow optimally.

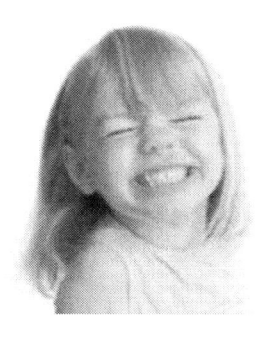 He showed this through images of tooth development in groups of people all over the world.

When groups of people who never had access to those foods came in contact with it, tooth decay & irregular bite occurred within one generation & nasal passage deformity became common.

If you have children, you obviously want the best for them.

Could the food you feed them affect the development of their faces, bodies & brains? The answer is most definitely yes.

Could these displacement foods, which are readily available to all of us in the Western world, be major players in obesity, the inability to lower body fat, a drop in mental & physical performance & many other health issues?

If you have never thought about it in this way before, now is the time to sit up & take stock.

What are displacement foods?

This term basically means that they use up more of your body's resources to digest than they provide. This will slowly drain your health "bank account" until you are in the red…or dead.

Sometimes, even when you choose a healthy option, like a piece of fruit, over a pack of sweets, that fruit can be so old it contains little nutrition. (However, it could still be your best choice.)

Ever bitten into an apple that looks shiny & bright, but is practically mush?

Large companies have been known to hold apples in factories for over a month. Spray them with wax so they look healthy & fresh & then release them into stores once the price of apples has gone up. Makes sense to maximise profits but…

How can this go on?

More importantly, what is the long-term effect of this behavior? It's not coincidence that this sort of practice runs smoothly alongside the rapid rise in obesity around the Western world.

Top Tip:
Eat organic whenever you can from a respected supplier.

This will make sure you are not ingesting any poisons that can, over time, affect your hormones, increase your body fat & negatively affect your physical & mental performance.

If…

If you don't have these two main points handled, then your body resorts to grabbing these toxins & storing them in fat away from your internal organs.

A vicious circle can develop, where you crave foods that make you fatter in order to have storage space for these toxins.

Your body is smart. It physically stores the danger to protect your vital organs. It cannot allow toxins to damage your organs, or your life expectancy will be reduced.

A state of extreme ill health arises when fat buildup is at an overflow point. The fat overflows from your surrounding body areas & begins to cake around your internal organs—& this is where disease really starts to rear its ugly head.

You should have a plan to support & improve your detoxification pathways, because fat loss unlocks toxins that need to leave your body. This is one factor that can hold a lot of people back from real fat-loss results.

They simply do not have enough antioxidants - molecules that clean your system of damage from oxidation, free radicals, that are a form of byproduct from everyday living or damage to tissue.

Nutritional support is essential. The last section of this book provides you with a system to improve your health status, vitamin & mineral levels, fitness levels & physical appearance through supplementation.

That last section underpins & supports the three sections before it. The four sections work hand-in-hand to boost your mental, physical & emotional performance—as well as drastically reshaping your physical appearance.

As you apply the principles within each section you will begin to notice a shift in your mental & physical state. After repeated efforts you will reach your optimal state of being where your body & brain function at their peak.

All that Stress

I spoke about stress in detail earlier, but it comes in again here. Applying yourself in a specific way against stress helps you lose fat.

You cannot avoid stress in the sense that you & everyone else experience it everyday in some form or another. The trick is to manage that process optimally.

Take responsibility for the fact that stress causes obesity—don't just chalk it up to bad eating or an unhealthy lifestyle alone. It is one piece of a large puzzle.

Here is a quick overview:

Your lifestyle, movements, eating habits, or external pollutants stress you. Your adrenals receive the signal from your pituitary gland to create more cortisol (stress hormone).

Overproduction of cortisol leads to inflammation in your gut & the death of healthy gut flora.

Your histamine levels (a chemical compound involved in regulating your immune system & function of your gut) also rise in response to this elevated cortisol. This leads to a more reactive digestive tract that makes you sensitive to foods—which in turn stresses you more.

This reaction disrupts your insulin receptor sites, resulting in a form of insulin intolerance. Your body then creates more insulin, as it cannot balance your blood-sugar levels optimally.

The extra insulin ages & damages your cells, creating more stress. This makes you crave foods that offer release from the pain/inflammation/stressful feeling but that also aggravate your gut, increase insulin production & sends you back to the start of this painful cycle.

It's up to you to break the cycle & get yourself out of this viscous circle & into a *virtuous circle* of upward spiraling positive events instead. This book can help you make that a reality.

All you have is this moment, this decision, no one ever at a doughnut by accident! You choose what to eat & when to eat it. With a little practice you will master your food choice at each meal & give yourself the best chance at optimal living.

If you are insanely stressed in a negative way, then there is every chance that you are on your way to serious fat gain – there are things you can do to prevent this...

Prevent it by using the methods outlined near the beginning & throughout this book. The systems & techniques I provide you will help you better manage the stress load that you encounter each day.

Malnutrition: Invisible Epidemic

The third of the early warning signs is malnutrition. I'll bet your mind instantly takes you to *National Geographic* images of starving kids in Africa. But that's not the only way malnutrition presents itself.

What if I told you that a lot of people in the western world are slowly starving to death?

A high percentage of the food that people eat these days does not contain enough nutrients for optimal vitality. It's simply high-energy, high-calorie food that causes a deep, unsettling hunger for more nourishment. However that craving is usually met with more empty-calorie food.

A lot of your cravings are your body desiring certain vitamins & minerals. You eat something & think you should be satisfied, but because the food you put in your stomach doesn't contain what your body needs, you're left wanting more,

Obese people are malnourished because they don't get the right nutrients from their poor diet. It's like running a car on vegetable oil instead of petrol. It may work, but won't perform optimally—or for long.

The main point is that eating food is not *only* about taste, desire, or pleasure—it's about *nourishment*. Your body needs to absorb essential nutrients in order to function optimally.

Most people eat food for its taste or for the fun or experience. This is absolutely fine, *if* you are well nourished & healthy.

However, if your vitamin & mineral levels are not at ideal levels, then eating for the experience alone is not for you.

Peak for Experience

Once you get to peak health & physical condition, then you can enjoy food purely for the taste. Any condition you find yourself in before that optimal state, then your food choices should be made based on vitality, health & function.

I am not saying that healthy food is not a tasty or enjoyable experience. Healthy food isn't a sugar rush or a bloated full feeling. The experience is different.

The problem is that most people go for the less healthy option more than the healthy food experience. Why is this?

Eat purely for taste, a full to the brim feeling & a rush sensation, or eat for health, vitality & a rush of content-ness within your body & mind. The choice is yours. The result of your choice is far-reaching.

Foods that are higher in nutrients can also be tasty. As mentioned earlier the marketing for processed sweetened & genetically modified food is aggressive & thorough. We cannot avoid it in the western world.

A good rule of thumb is to only eat occasionally or never at all a food that has a marketing campaign behind it. Reason being that it likely has been genetically altered or processed in some way & therefore requires aggressive selling to make profit.

If you are used to eating a sweet diet, pastries, breads, chocolate, sweets, desserts & sugared tea or coffee then as you first switch to lower GI foods (the release of their energy into your bloodstream is slower) it may take a week or so for your taste buds to adjust back from the sweetened, salty, or fatty foods that you might be used to.

This is because lower GI foods are in general less sweet of a sensation on your taste buds. There is also reaction going on within your body & mind, the difference in response of your body to a high GI meal compared to a low GI meal is dramatic.

The lower GI meal will cause less stress on your system.

As the average person eats 2-3 meals a day this is a high volume stressor day after day that can ultimately be managed by you.

After about 7-10 days of adjustment on to the lower GI choice foods, the 'sweet tooth' person will find the healthier food options (lower GI in this case) just as tasty—or even more so.

Often people who initially resist cutting out certain foods & replacing them with others will start saying things like, "I had steak & vegetables the other night & it was *so* tasty!" This taste bud transition can happen in a short space of time.

They'll also make comments such as, "I ate a chocolate bar (or another favorite sweet) & it tasted so synthetic, like I was eating sweet plastic."

As you improve your health & vitality you will become more sensitive to the taste of the food you eat & the affect it has on your body & mind. This will in time strengthen your food choices toward the healthy option.

Principle Exercise 15
You Are What You Eat MyFitPal

- *Download the MyFitnessPal app from the app store onto your phone or computer.*

- *Set up an account.*

Important—Pay Attention!*

Daily Calorie Intake

- *On the top-left corner of your Diary page is Goal (calories).*

- *You can alter this figure within the settings:*

  - *Press More (bottom right),*

  - *Then Goals, then adjust the calorie section to the suggested figure below.*

- *This amount can fluctuate depending on your activity level & state of health.*

- *At the time of writing, for the average person to maintain weight the NHS provides these guidlelines:*

2500kcal for men[1]

2000 kcal for women[1]

---

1 http://www.nhs.uk/chq/pages/1126.aspx?categoryid=51

This figure may not be optimal for everyone. Some factors that can alter your calorie requirements are age, lifestyle, height & weight, hormone balance, medications & level of health.

I have found that the following calorie variable works best for most people. Please note this figure requires regular adjustment & should be used as a guideline for the purpose of this example.

For accurate adjustment seek a qualified professional.

Men: 1700–2500 calories per day.

Women: 1300–1900 calories per day.

You must consume enough calories every day—for example 2000 (men) & 1500 (women).

**You must not consistently under eat.
This is a strict rule that you must adhere to.**

A very important point to consider is the source of your calories.

The type of food – organic / non-organic, processed, gmo, high fat, carb or protein content. I'll provide you with a list of foods that studies show & I have found to be the wisest choice if you want to remain in a consistent state of optimal health.

Your food counter should look similar to this:

If you consistently undereat, it's just a matter of time before you fall ill or sustain an injury.

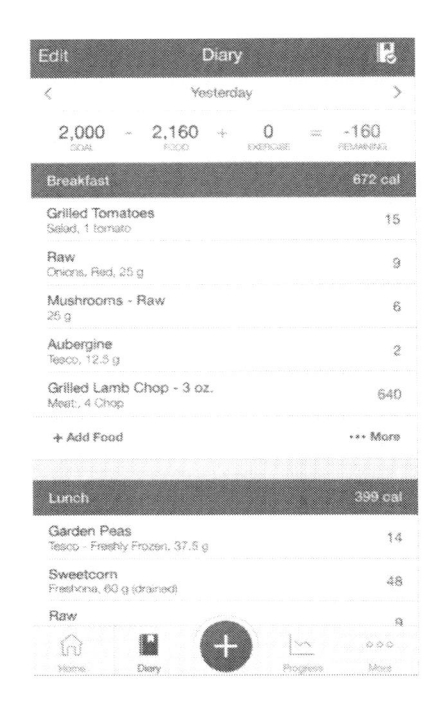

I have seen this many times.

In addition, this obviously puts a stop to your ShapeTraining.

Here's an example of a man's food diary.

Pay particular attention to the top left figures for Goal & Food u

Steps

Macronutrient intake

- *Your calorie intake will be segmented into macronutrients: protein, carbohydrates (carbs) & fats.*

- *Which macronutrient provides the bulk of your energy/calories for each day is one of the keys to optimal heath & fitness.*

To see an image of your daily macronutrient intake press:

- On the diary screen press the top left button calorie figure (goal).

*- Alternatively press 'More' (bottom right)—
Nutrition—A pie chart image will appear. This is a
great visual to see exactly what macronutrients are
providing your energy that day.*

For your daily intake, reach approximations of:

- *50 percent protein*

—This is essential.

- **30 percent fat (this will need adjustment over time
with the help of a health care professional but this gives
you a baseline figure that you can always revert to)**

**20 percent carbohydrates (This will also need adjustment
over time especially around specific sporting events or unique
requirements, but for now this acts as a good starting figure)**

Here is an image of what you should see:

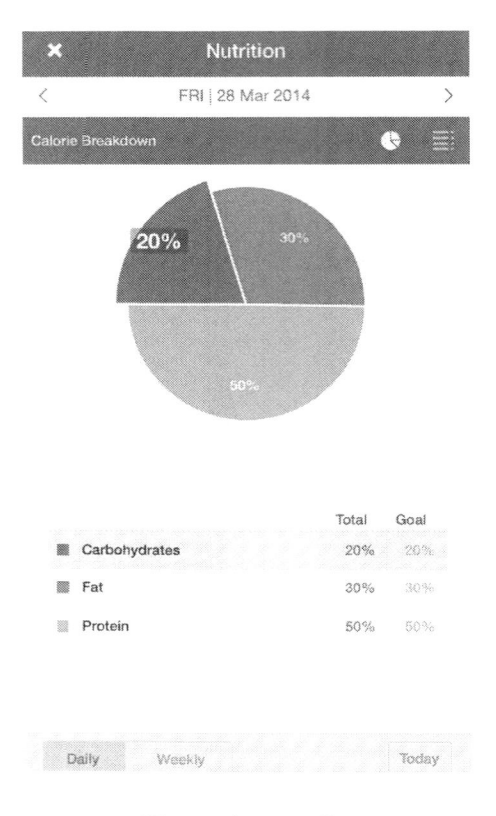

*Protein goal—
Important. Pay attention!*

Protein

- *Aim to consume: Men: three times your weight in kilograms of bodyweight per day in grams of protein.*

Women: twice your weight in kilograms per day in grams of protein.

- *Example: 80kg (176lbs) man = 240 grams of protein per day.*

You can keep an eye on this from the diary screen, press:

Top left calorie figure (GOAL)— this will take you to the pie chart image – now press the lines underneath the top right hand corner arrow. – You will now see a data view of your daily food intake. This data lists your intake in grams.

- **Your food choice will have an affect on your data & therefore different effects on your body composition, state of health & performance levels.**

- *The longer you use this app, the more aware you will become about what foods bring about a healthier, happier you. Eventually you will make wise food choices without the need for an app – but until you truly understand this process use the app & the information I provide you here.*

Carbs

- *It takes approximately twenty-one to twenty-eight days to turn your body to a fat adapter.*

- *This means your body will choose to burn fat as a fuel more quickly than it does at present.*

- *Once this happens, you'll find it much easier to burn fat, get lean & looked ripped.*

The way to make this happen is to keep your carb intake low for up to four weeks.

I advise my clients to eat no more than one hundred grams of carbohydrates per day for up to twenty-eight days.

- To keep a close eye on your carb intake, from the diary screen, press:

Top left calorie figure (GOAL)— this will take you to the pie chart image – now press the lines underneath the top right hand corner arrow. – You will now see a data view of your daily food intake. This data lists your intake in grams.

- *Look for 'Total Carbohydrates (g)'.*

Keep that figure below one hundred. You do that by controlling the amount of carbohydrates you eat.

You can consume even fewer grams of carbs per day than 100 for a while. This will eventually help you to become Insulin sensitive & 'carb tolerant'. Meaning you will be able to eat more carbs without negative effect. Over time this amount should be altered depending on your state of health & goal.

- *The type of carbs you eat is determined by your "Food Shopping List," which we'll go through shortly.*

Fat

- *For most people, approximately 75 percent of the population, it is a healthier approach to consume more 'good fats' than more carbs.*

- *The quality of fat is critically important.*

- *Ideally, fats should come from virgin coconut oil, olive oil & organic butter.*

- *Nuts & avocados can also be incorporated as good, healthy fats.*

- *Tweak a meal or two to perfect your calorie intake, keeping your macronutrient chart proportions in mind.*

Remember your macronutrients are protein, fat & carbs. I have provided you the guidelines.

• *Play with this. The more you use the app, the more you'll understand what works best for you & how one food choice at one meal can affect your entire day negatively.*

Principle 15
I Eat For Optimal Health & Performance

In order to reach optimal health & fitness, you must learn how to fuel your health & your inevitable success.

My system has been tried & tested by hundreds of people to great effect.

After approximately seven weeks, you will feel leaner, stronger, fitter, mentally sharper, more energetic & healthier.

The system I have provided you above will teach you how to eat for health, performance & taste rather than just for taste.

Once you learn this, you will never be able to unlearn it.

This is a "pure gem" on your road to optimal health & fitness.

This is one of the master keys that will open many doors for you on your road to even greater success.

You Get to Choose

If you keep putting lots of high-calorie foods into your mouth with little—or even zero—nutritional value, you will eventually slip into obesity, disease & dysfunction.

You may get away with it for a while—for some, it's many years—but eventually it will catch up with you!

When you lack nutrients, your body snaps into a state of deficiency. You will feel hungry all the time, tired, unable to focus, unable to motivate yourself & have a poor sex drive that could cause problems in your relationship or with your self-esteem.

Everything falls apart when your health bank account dips into negative figures.

- The solution to this is to send the pendulum in the opposite direction. Eat for health, eat for nutrients—& eat for more life.

- Enjoy the taste of the foods you *can* eat. Nutrition is the fastest way to reshape your body for the long-term & get the most enjoyment out of life, because when you eat this way you are vital & healthy enough to truly enjoy it.

- The simple answer is to eat the food that we have evolved to burn as fuel. We'll go into this in some detail within this chapter.

Assess Your Nutrition

It is vital that you are honest in this section, because it will form the basis of the diet you'll switch to in the coming days & weeks.

Answer these questions & take the actions suggested:

- What types of food do you eat on a day-to-day basis? Processed or fresh organic? Sweet or savoury? Etc.

- Score your percentage of carbohydrates, protein & fats. MyFitnessPal is a great app/website for this. It's free & calculates everything for you. You just have to input the foods you eat. Be conscious of which macronutrient provides the bulk of your daily calorie intake.

- How do you feel after each meal? Write down, in detail, how you feel after each meal. Use notes in your phone to make it easy & accessible.

- How do you feel, in general, after eating or throughout your day? For instance do you always have a dip of energy & focus around 2pm?

- How large are your portion sizes? Become aware of how much or how little you are eating in comparison to others. Using the guidelines I have provided through MyFitnessPal will determine the quantity of food you eat through the day. How you spread that amount out will be your choice.

- Would you say you overeat? You should be able to explain & justify your answer.

- Do you constantly feel hungry? If so, why do you think that is?

- Describe your hunger pain. This helps to understand it. Sometimes it isn't actually hunger, it can be dehydration for instance. Or there could be some mental unrest from a psychological perspective that causes you to feel like you are hungry all the time. Simply become aware of your hunger right now.

- What do you think is your ideal weight? Talk with your health care professional & friends to see if they agree with you. I know it is easily said, but do not obsess over your weight. You would be wiser to focus on your body-fat percentage & set goals from that perspective. The BioSignature system is perfect for this. I will introduce you to this as you read on.

- Do you find it hard to lose fat if you try?

- How do you feel about food? Do you love to eat, or can you take it or leave it?

- Do you suffer from food cravings?

- List the foods you crave the most.

- How often do you eat what you consider to be a really healthy meal?

- Would you describe yourself as "malnourished?" You should be able to explain your answer.

Dicing With Your Health…

Nutrition is a dicey subject. Some "online diet experts" believe that you can eat anything as long as your calories are low. This line of thinking does not take physical fitness or your long-term health into account—only fat or weight loss.

You should look at the bigger picture if you want long-lasting results.

Without the nutrients, you won't be able to build muscle fast, or enjoy rapid fat loss from the places that matter & remain healthy for long. On top of which, as you go through this process you will likely not be able to perform at your peak.

I can teach you a way to optimilise your body-fat while functioning at your peak. When you start to live by the principles within this book that is the natural state you will take.

Spend some time answering the questions above to get a better idea of how you relate to food, both consciously and unconsciously. Simply become more aware of your current state.

Many of my clients are horrified when they realise how badly they eat because of their busy, stressful & high-pressure lifestyles.

This is often missed. I get them to fill in their food diary & we look at the data. A lot of people don't realise how many carbohydrates they eat on a day-to-day basis.

Sometimes a person sees that 75 percent of the daily calories came from fat & only 10 percent from protein! While this may be ok for a day or two it will certainly become a problem over time. Inability to control body-fat stores will be one of the issues.

All these situations can be easily corrected with a little planning & preparation. In the long run, it's worth it for the extra energy & zest of life that comes from these positive changes.

Talking about the general population, what most find is that when they tweak their diet, they find they're less bloated & that their belly shrinks dramatically, like deflating a balloon.

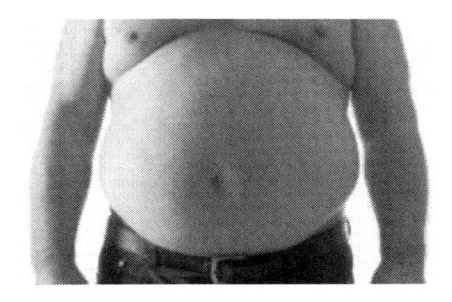

The problem with bad food choices is not only a lack of nutrients, but the aggravation this causes in your stomach & intestines.

This inflammation can also be a massive block to fat loss. As explained earlier, you'll see how this fits into the vicious cycle of fat gain through stress.

Reduce Inflammation like the Boss

Nutrients are like nature's medicine & they each have specific reactions in the human body.

One of the best things about healthy food is that it naturally reduces inflammation—& inflammation is a solid building block for some of the biggest, scariest diseases of our time.

When you keep your body healthy & don't inspire a climate of constant inflammation, you won't go through the pain, worry & illness that result from chronic disease, disorder & depression.

Chronic inflammation is always present in obese individuals. That is why so many *fat* people find it hard to eat healthy. They are most certainly fat & depressed.

The constant aggravation in their guts fuels a fire that needs feeding. This reduces absorption of vital nutrients & creates food cravings.

The end result is usually diabetes with a supporting cast of disorders & deficiencies.

Here are a few food tips to reverse these effects & restore your health & wellness:

- **Fresh food**
  Food that has not been coupled with other foods, or been turned into a "product" are better for your body. Think about it like this: If it wasn't available 10,000 years ago don't eat it.

- **Genetically Modified Organisms (GMOs)**
  GMO foods are foods that have been genetically modified by man. As no one knows the true outcome of eating these foods, this is one of the biggest experiments with human health the world has ever seen. Do you want to be a subject of it?

  Read food labels & source good restaurants who serve fresh quality produce. Nowadays it is very hard to avoid GMO but make a conscious effort to stop those foods entering your body. No one ever at a tomato by accident... or a doughnut for that matter!

- **Fresh fruit & vegetables**
  When these foods are fresh they are jam packed with goodness. These foods pump your body full of nutrients. The more you eat, the better you'll feel.

  Fruit is good for you, but—like everything else— only in moderation. If you know you're fat right now, then a week off fruit (& all sugars) would likely do you good. Eat as many green vegetables as you can instead as they will not negatively affect your body composition or health.

  Source fresh organic fruit & vegetables whenever you can. Farmers markets can be great for this. Nowadays there are many options on organic delivery of these foods so you can steer well clear of 'made for maximum profit' supermarket options.

Take the time to source a respected trusted supplier or have someone reliable do the research for you – it is worth it.

- *Eat more protein.*
  Most people don't eat enough protein. This leads to an inability to lose weight, poor health & an inability to put on muscle. The first sixty grams of protein you eat goes to your immune system & detoxification.

  You can only grow more muscle or build quality tissue after that. If you don't get this much, then you shortchange yourself & dramatically decrease your chances of success & happiness.

- *Change your mind-set.*
  The cereal for breakfast, sandwich for lunch, potatoes for dinner mind-set every day of your life leaves you with a carb-heavy meal at every sitting. Lose the cereal, bread & potatoes & make *variety* your new mantra. Use the food list that appears later to make up your meals.

- *Eat two different vegetables every meal.*
  Try this at every meal until you have exhausted your options & then start back at the beginning of the list. Keep this up. It will provide you with essential fiber, a variety of nutrients & health-giving properties.

- *Do not eat sugar.*

Also don't eat high-carbohydrate foods in any way, shape, or form. The glycemic index of the food (how fast the energy of the food is released into your bloodstream) should determine your food choices if health & performance are of concern.

I will provide you with a food list to choose from that gives you a selection of 'low GI' foods to choose from. This list is extensive so do not be concerned about restrictive eating.

High carb foods, like sweets, doughnuts, pastries & the like poison your body—full stop. Processed food & fast food should be a joke to you—you may as well be eating disease & saying, "Diabetes, bring it on."

- **Use lemon & lime in your water.**
  This will alkalize your internal system & turn down the acidity of your digestive tract[1]

Consuming these juices will help put out the fire that is likely raging within your gut – this fire is raging for most people these days.

Because of the low sugar content & high alkaline mineral content lemon & limes have an alkalizing affect on the body even though they are an acidic food with a pH of around 2.

Once you help to extinguish this fire your health, vitality & performance will all increase.

---

1 http://www.energiseforlife.com/wordpress/2010/08/18/alkaline-water-lemon-water-is-alkaline-an-explanation/

While lemons & limes provide approximately the same amount of citric acid per gram, lemon will provide a little more sugar than lime.

Personally I prefer limes to lemons but either will do a good job in decreasing acid conditions within your intestinal tract – a very good thing in this day & age.

Lime juice can also kill off certain bacterial strains helping to lower your bacterial load therefore leaving you with more energy to use elsewhere[2].

- **Fish oil.**
  One of the best supplements you could invest in. On top of calming inflammation like a hose on a fire, it has an endless list of beneficial properties. More about this later…

One effective way to control inflammation is through nutrition by cutting out foods that stimulate the fire & introducing a range of healthy foods that actively restore your body's natural healing processes.

You likely already realised that pizzas, burgers, chips & sweets caused inflammation in your body—creating the ideal climate for *more* fat gain & disease – now is the time to kick them out of your diet for good.

The Good/Cheat Dilemma

The word *diet* originates from the Greek word for "way of life." However, our society heavily associates it with restriction.

Your personal diet—way of life—should bring about optimal health & fitness that is a simple, natural, everyday occurrence.

---

2 http://www.ncbi.nlm.nih.gov/pubmed/7501870

The *big* secret that no one talks about is that eating "junk"—empty calories—makes you crave junkier, emptier calories. It's a vicious circle.

When you break this cycle & feed your body healthy food instead, you recover, improve & enrich your life experiences.

- If I offered you a *free* food item to eat every day that was absolutely delicious, but guaranteed that you would become obese & riddled with disease in a few short years, I bet you would *not* eat it.

- But this is what's going on all around us. Buy one get one free or super cheap food. Do you think that a burger that costs two dollars or one pound could do you *any good at all?* In fact, it is most certainly doing you harm.

- Yet this is exactly what people do when they eat varieties of processed, refined, sugar-laden junk food with little-to-zero nutrients.

- It may be cheap, it may even taste good, but it's draining your "health bank account"—*fast.*

This makes the concept of a treat ridiculous! It implies that you are "treating" yourself to the thing that makes you ill—the poor quality food. You're treating your self to disease.

Change your mind-set & embrace the idea that you have been cheating yourself by eating that junk—this simple shift will help you dramatically over time.

Healthy food is natural. It's what you were born to eat & what healthy populations have thrived on for millions of years.

The moment industry took off & poor quality food became widely available, tooth decay became more common & facial spacing was disrupted as illustrated by Western A Price in his book Nutrition and Physical Degeneration.

Price found that within one generation of consumption of 'white man food' (bleached white rice, white bread & white sugar) that babies where being born with palate & facial abnormalities. More & more children required braces.[2]

He documents this visually by taking many photos of the alterations in facial structure. The parents of these children & their parents did not have trouble with tooth decay, palate or facial misalignment.

Could the consumption of the 'white man' food cause a form of malnutrition within the person that stunts perfect growth & formation of bony structures?

In a more recent study into facial abnormalities within the Proceedings of the National Academy of Sciences, Noreen von Cramon-Taubadel hypothesised that facial structure altered as the generation transitioned from hunter-gatherers to farmers.[1]

Postindustrial populations have more experience of the orthodontist's chair[2]. This is a growing industry. Could this be partly due to the decrease in nutrition within the western worlds food supply due to increased sales of processed & fast foods?[3]

It is no coincidence that we are unhealthier today than ever before in human history.

---

2 Nutrition and Physical Degeneration by Western A Price.

1 http://www.pnas.org/search?fulltext=Noreen+von+Cramon-Taubadel&submit=yes&x=0&y=0

2 http://www.strategyr.com/Orthodontic_Supplies_Market_Report.asp

3 http://www.statista.com/topics/863/fast-food/

Creating optimal health is about feeding your body the nutrients it needs. If you want to snack on something that's not ideal for your health & vitality every now & then, fine. This will not kill (well not instantly anyway).

The real problems arrive when you consume low nutrient food daily. A muffin, processed bread, cereal, fast food meals etc. etc.

This type of eating is a reality these days & a very common one. The trick is to avoid the invisibly dangerous, widely consumed food products that cause physical degeneration in people on a regular basis – low nutrient highly processed food.

When you avoid these foods you will become more aware of how each meal makes you feel & start to make choices based on health & taste, rather than taste alone.

You can make healthy desserts & snacks that look & taste like you are "treating yourself" when you are, in fact, taking in more vital nutrients.

This is the way to live. This is the way to truly enjoy your life, through a vital & vibrant body & mind.

Over time, eating in a healthy manner will change the taste you experience on your palate. You'll find healthy foods tastier than ever before.

If you eat in a highly nutritious way throughout your life then you can affect your child's facial alignment as demonstrated by Western A Price. So if eating in a healthy way to feel more vital & experience more energy is not enough of an incentive for you, then think about your future children & how you could help them – starting now.

Chapter 10:
Nourish Now or Pay the Price

The healthy man is the thin man. But you don't need to go hungry for it: Remove the flours, starches & sugars; that's all.

—*Samael Aun Weor*
Author, lecturer & Founder of the Universal
Christian Gnostic

I have never met anyone who doesn't have a complicated relationship with food, The act of eating & the pleasure or displeasure people get from eating, can become dysfunctional if thought about too much.

You need nutrition to thrive & now is the moment to concede that—not tomorrow, not next week & not after one last pizza. Right now.

In the future, you'll thank your present self for making the positive change quickly.

Are You Eating these Wellness Foods?

You may remember in school when the teacher showed you the food pyramid & taught you briefly about each macronutrient & its role in your body.

Back then, they taught us that eating high-carb foods was good for us. Ouch! In the most part – approximately 75 percent of the population –are carb intolerant. Meaning they do not need to eat as much carbohydrate as they currently consume.

Things have changed now. New scientific studies are being published all the time proving that the opposite is true. You can turn the old model of the food pyramid upside down to a healthier impression of the way you should be eating – if health, vitality & freedom from disease are important to you.

The amount of carbohydrate requirement varies for each individual. Part of your job is to determine how much is perfect for you. The amount may fluctuate from week to week due to your daily requirements & the chemistry of your body.

However, you can figure out a ballpark figure that you can follow on a day-to-day basis. This is the best course of action for your long-term health.

You may also be in the 25 percent population—those who *are* carb tolerant. This means you can eat more carbohydrates than others without as much negative effect.

One easy way to tell is from your body shape. You have insulin receptor sites located around your body. When you consume too many carbohydrates, you'll lay down more fat at these locations.

The reason is that when you eat carbs, your body produces more insulin to balance your blood-sugar level. When this happens en masse, your insulin sites respond in a form of swelling or activity.

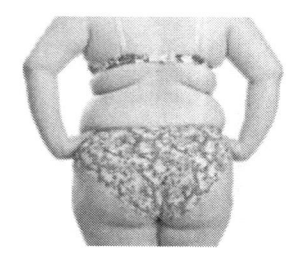

One insulin site is directly above your hip bones, a second is just under your shoulder blades.

When you gain fat in these areas, you know you're eating more carbs than what you really need.

And, yes, when you reduce your carb intake, these areas get thinner.

Your body is a system of interconnected systems. When you improve one area, many other areas of your body also improve (& vice versa).

Quick Tips:

- *Eat lots of vegetables*
  Eat them like most people currently eat potatoes, fries, chips, rice, pasta, bread—all carbohydrates. Vegetables, particularly the green ones, are low GI, meaning they will not affect your blood sugar level so intensely. They also provide a number of other health benefits, I will expand on these as you read on.

- *Watch your fruit intake*
  Certain fruits are high in natural sugars & vitamins. There's a perfect amount of fruit you should eat every day. It may be one piece, or it may be five. It mostly depends on your carb tolerance & activity levels. My system will help you determine this amount. Otherwise a good nutritionist or qualified health professional should be able to guide you.

- *Consume high-quality sources of protein*
  Free-range, organic meat helps build solid muscle, repair & build bone & also keep your immune system functioning optimally. The less chemicals in your protein, the less your body has to work to process that junk out of your system.

- *Moderate amounts, or zero, dairy*
  If you're dairy intolerant, then you should avoid it at all times. A food-intolerance test will determine this for you. People commonly have intolerance to dairy for many years, but the symptoms are so subtle they never notice. They can never figure out why they still have a bloated belly. Get tested to be sure. If you're

in or around the London UK area you can book this through my website.

- *Some, or zero, whole grains*
  The wise choice would be to eat these occasionally & not much of them. However, the food-intolerance test will confirm if it's wise for you to consume this food type at all.

- *Drink plenty of clean water daily*
  This is important so your body can detox effectively. If you want clear skin, sparkling eyes & healthy, shiny hair, drink quality liquid every day. Most people miss the connection between water intake & energy levels. Optimal clean water in take can increase productivity.[1], [2]

- *Add nuts, berries & green leaves to your diet*
  Eat the way nature intended. Your body & brain will then serve you well. A warning with the nut intake— again, it's best to determine any intolerance or allergy to nuts before you start gorging on them. Get a food-intolerance test. Source a reliable test through your health care professional. I have a system in place for my clients in London, you can check out this system through my website –12 Week Supplementation Program (12WSP).

Does Your Diet Match Up?

---

1 http://www.ncbi.nlm.nih.gov/pubmed/20974676

2 http://www.naturalhydrationcouncil.org.uk/wp-content/uploads/2012/06/Hydration-at-Work.pdf

Most people when they take a look at what they eat, probably find that not only are carbohydrates the dominating macronutrient of their diet, but they're also the *only* part they care about getting enough of.

This is because these types of food are heavily marketed on a daily basis. The big food companies that sell these products do their jobs effectively.

Their job is to sell more of their product to as many people as possible. If they can smear other competing products, like healthy organic food, to make theirs look better, of course they will.

So be aware of information in the media that rubbish the benefits of organic, free range food. It is likely this type of information was funded by a processed food company.

On top of this, processed carb foods are cheaper & easier to prepare, so this alone makes them more appealing to the fast paced lifestyles of most of us today.

However, like with an investment portfolio you must think long-term investment while at the same time as having some short-term returns. What I mean is, do not eat purely for short term satisfaction, you must think long-term about your health & this means eating healthy meals 9 out 10 meal sittings.

Cheap as Chips

I've seen meals in fast-food restaurants for less than three pounds or four dollars. How can an organically grown vegetable & grass-fed fillet steak compete with that price?

If you eat based on price, you're heading down a dark road. Food is the most important investment of your life. From a business perspective, would you keep putting your money into cheap products that eventually caused harm to your consumers?

This is obviously not a good business model—it's not a good health model either.

Easy Is Not Always Best

No doubt you are time poor—most people are these days. If you don't take the time to prepare yourself healthy meals or have someone prepare them for you, then you will soon become *health poor*—and then you'll have lots of time on your hands, but you'll be unable to do anything constructive with it.

Processed meals & refined carbs are definitely easier to prepare than most healthy meals, although the positives of decreased prep time are dramatically overshadowed by the lack of nutrients.

Right now the average persons diet looks like this:

- Bread, pasta, rice, baked goods (processed white carbs)

- Cakes, sweets, chocolate, store-bought sauces (sugar)

- Junk food when you don't have time to cook

- A little protein to go with your carbohydrates

- A smattering of vegetables or fruit because you "have to" eat them.

If you eat like an average person then you will be an average person. I can guess that you do not want that status for yourself. I presume that you would much prefer to be outstanding rather than average.

The modern Western diet is based on the grocery-store model of sales—"instant is better." Of course, you sacrifice health when you want instant food.

Microwave meals, boxed meals, store sauces—even foods you deem "healthy" all contain sugar, preservatives, monosodium glutamate & many other harmful toxins.

Monosodium glutamate is a naturally occurring salt from the amino acid glutamic acid. Although past safe by the food & drug administration (FDA) many people have reported adverse effects from eating it. It is well known that it is added to some Chinese take-away cuisine & canned foods.

If you eat processed, pre-made, ready meals & most packaged food from the store then the bulk of your diet will contain toxins & simple sugars.

You need to regularly adjust your eating patterns if you are going to achieve a level of health & wellness that will help you build a powerful super-fit body & mind.

Ideally you should eat organic food that is free of toxins, grown naturally & intended to give your body nutrients & health, *rather than* non-organic food that is mass-produced to last longer on the shelves, where profit is the source of its creation.

Principle Exercise 16
Know What You Eat

This exercise will increase your awareness around the quality of the food that you choose to eat.

Look at it this way; Imagine a business bank account, one where you are charged for every deposit. The size of the deposit is irrelevant but for some deposits you are charged £2 or $2, for other types of deposit you are charged £5 or $5 & for another type of deposit you are charged £10 or $10.

Now if you're wise you will channel your deposits in through the route that deducts the least from your money & you'll aim to have the deposits be as large as possible. Simple right, stay with me here.

At this point understand that when you eat a food it takes energy & enzymes to digest that food. Some foods take more energy & enzymes than others. Some foods provide more nutrients than others.

Now some foods provide very little nutrients (a tiny deposit of money), while at the same time require enzymes & energy in order to be processed by your body (£10 or $10 fee).

Imagine at this point if you choose to eat these foods all the time, at every meal, year after year. What would your bank account look like? – Not that healthy, right!

This is the choice you make with your level of health each time you eat a food & a meal. Make a smart choice & you boost your health bank account, make an ignorant choice & you slowly but surely drain your health account.

Write down what you eat today. You can look at this in the digital food diary
I introduced you to earlier.

Become aware of what you usually eat in any given week.
Notice if you eat a lot of one particular food.
Is that food a healthy food? Be honest.

Do some research on what the nutritional values are of the foods you eat regularly.

Also note the extra ingredients you eat that you may not have been aware of. These are things like; high fructose corn syrup, wheat, gluten, artificial flavours & colourings etc.

The above list are commonly within ready meals, TV dinners & processed foods.
Look at the labels. Avoid the bad stuff. It matters.

Principle 16
I Purposefully Choose Vitality Food For Every Meal

Some foods increase your vitality, some foods decrease it. Vitality foods are nutrient dense foods that you are not intolerant or allergic to.

Become aware of the food you eat & why you choose to eat it. At your next meal ask yourself 'Why do I feel like eating that type of food today?'

From the information provided to you so far, you'll begin to understand the effect each food choice & meal will have on your body & mind, both short-term & long-term.

Over time, these elements are part of what determines your level of success. Your food choices can either hold you back or drive you forward. It is one of the things that you have full control over in your life.

If you feel that you do not have control over your food choices then it is time to seek some coaching. Get some structured powerful techniques in place so that you own your food choices & therefore control the direction & shape of your body & life.

Begin to make more educated, smarter choices for every meal of every day, week after week.

Once you live with this principle, in a short space of time, you will notice a subtle shift in your energy levels & thought patterns – for the better.

Eating foods that are lower or free from chemical cocktails means those chemicals are not swimming around your blood stream affecting your muscle, bones, internal organs & brain.

The less time your body has to spend on getting rid of these chemicals the more time it can spend on growing.

The High-Protein Plan

Let's talk about increasing your protein intake at every meal. Back in caveman days, meat was consumed liberally when hunts were successful.

Of course, cavemen also had to physically catch their protein back then. The rest of the time, they lived off berries, nuts, fruits & things that grew in the ground.

A big part of Optimalism is realising that you need adequate amounts of protein to reach optimal health.

Why protein? In order to detoxify optimally you require protein, in order for your immune system to function optimally you require appropriate amounts of protein, in order to grow, repair & form new cells you require a certain amount of protein.

It is different forms of protein that are required at different stages of each process & the requirements depend heavily on what area of your body requires it.

For instance amino acids are required in varying amounts to detoxify & grow more muscle. Collagen is another form of protein that is required for hardening of bones & proper bone formation.

In order for your immune system to function at maximum capacity it requires regular doses of protein. Immunoglobulins, also known as antibodies, are proteins that circulate in the blood, fight bacteria & support other proteins in immune function.

In order to make & keep, muscle (protein synthesis) you must consume appropriate amounts of protein. Your muscles are made of a selection of the macronutrients that you eat—protein, carbs & fat.

Protein makes up the bulk of the requirement needed to create adequate amounts of bone, tissue & muscle.

You are, literally, what you eat. So, if 50 percent of your calories come from fat, well, what would you expect to look like?

Protein helps build muscle, maintains it & facilitates fat loss. It is essential for detoxification, which, as we have talked about, is critical.

The first thirty grams of protein you eat goes purely toward detoxification. The second thirty grams goes to your immune system. The next thirty grams goes to repair & growth of tissue.

Without argument, you must consume a bare minimum of ninety grams of protein every day. The bigger you are, the more you need to consume to reach & remain at, optimal health.

If you play a sport, are active throughout your day, go to the gym or are unwell then you will require a higher protein intake.

A Protein Goal:

Male: 3.5 (Daily range of 3–4.3) grams of protein per kilogram of body weight.

Example: A man weighing100 kg should consume 350 grams of protein every day.

Female: 2 (Daily range of 2–2.5) grams of protein per kilogram of body weight.

Example: A 60-kg women should consume 120grams of protein every day.

You can easily monitor this by using MyFitnessPal, as explained earlier.

Immunity or Not to Be...

Most of your immune system—75 percent—is in your gut. You must consume adequate amounts of protein in order to heal tissue, fend off bacteria, fight disease & keep your gut healthy.

If you eat foods that damage your gut—low-quality food, foods you are intolerant to, or due to low gut health parasites manage to enter your system—then your gut will suffer injury & so will the rest of your body.

If your gut is injured, then so is your immune system. If your immune system is compromised, so will your strength be, both mental & physical strength.

The stronger your immune system is, the stronger you will be in the gym & throughout your life.

How strong you are physically, is directly related to the health of your immune system. If you want to feel stronger & perform better in the gym or at your chosen sport, boost your immune system. One surefire way is to increase your *protein intake (provided the source of protein is of good quality as talked about earlier).*

Not only does protein rebuild & reshape your body, it helps you become stronger across the board. *But* it's not just about the amount of protein you eat; it's also about the frequency that you eat it & the quality.

In My Opinion:

- *Eating some protein at every meal* is essential for optimum health.

- *Eating free-range, grass-fed animals* & *not* battery-caged animals that are pumped full of antibiotics, growth hormones & fed on GMO crops is a safer, long-term more effective strategy.

Solving The Low Carb Low Energy Problem...

You may have heard, or experienced yourself, that when you start a lower-carb, higher-protein diet, your energy levels can drop after a few days.

This in most cases is due to insufficient calorie intake. If you follow the guidelines I have provided you from Principle 14: Eat For Optimal Health & Fitness - you will not experience a drop in energy due to insufficient calorie intake.

Another reason energy levels can drop is a sudden decrease in sodium levels due to the digestion of the denser meats that you are now consuming.

Salt (sodium chloride) is required for the digestion & absorption of protein within your digestive tract. It is also heavily involved in the communication between you cells. The more protein you consume the more salt you require to maintain an optimal digestive process & cell communication.

Bear in mind that if you have high blood pressure then liberally salting your food may do you more harm than good – make sure you are aware of your blood pressure before piling the salt onto your next meal. However, for most people a little 'quality' salt will make an improvement to the meal & their energy levels.

Again I bring your attention to the quality of the food source, standard table salt has a very different nutritional quality to sea salt. Spend the few extra pennies & give yourself the best. Avoid standard table salt it's a chemical that you can do without.

Focus On Adding Rather Than Taking Away...

Most people think of a low carb diet as just removing those foods from their daily intake & going without. What I would prefer you to do is replace them with something else—which should in translation mean increased protein intake.

Focus on your protein goal for the day spreading your total gram figure across your meals for each day. So for example if you are a 60kg women then your protein goal should be 120grams of protein. If you plan to eat four meals today that means you need to get 30grams of protein into each meal. This amount of protein is approximately one to one & half chicken breasts.

Focusing on your calorie goal & your protein goal makes it much easier to forget about the carbs.

To clarify, if you are sensitive to your body's needs, you'll notice that the more protein you eat, the more your body needs salt. This is because sodium helps break down protein in your body & facilitates the communication between your cells.

As mentioned before feel free to add a little extra salt to things when you first start out.

The quality & quantity matters...

Your salt should be organic sea salt. Himalayan or Celtic are great sources & well worth the extra cost.

Fibre

If you were to cut carbs from you diet all together, you will at the same time cut two things that are essential for optimal health & fitness:

1. Fibre
2. Antioxidants

Therefore you may also need to add fibre to your diet as you maintain a lower carb intake for a period of time. High-protein diets can result in constipation if you don't eat enough vegetables with each meal.

Occasionally people experience slower bowel movements when they increase their protein & lower their carbs. This is a common issue that can be rectified easily. One simple way is to use fibre supplements.

A high protein & fat diet in the absence of fibre will result in endotoxemia (toxins on the walls of your cells which essential increase bacterial load) – this is a bad thing.

Some sources of supplemental fibre:

Psyllium husk

Linseeds

Potato Starch

Primal Fiber 1, 2 & 3 (available through my website)

Pop into your local health store & they will be able to assist you with fiber supplements. They are cheap & easy to implement into your routine.

When you get your fibre intake right, you'll notice your bowel movements are easier, more frequent (great for detoxifying) & more pleasurable.

On top of helping you go regularly, fibre is essential for proper illumination of xenoestrogens (foreign chemicals) & blood-sugar management.

By now, you are acutely aware of the importance of managing your blood-sugar levels. This is essential if you want low body fat & maintain a *high-health* status for the long-term.

Figuring Out the Fibre

Dietary fibre is an important part of a healthy diet. When you stop eating huge amounts of carbohydrates, you may not eat enough fibre. This is especially true when your protein intake increases.

You may need to "figure out the fibre" so that your digestive system runs smoothly. Basically there are two forms of fibre—soluble & insoluble.

Soluble fibres attract water & form a gel, which slows down digestion. Soluble fibre delays the emptying of your stomach & makes you feel full, which helps maintain appropriate portion control & satiety (feeling full & satisfied).

Slower stomach emptying may also affect blood-sugar levels & have a beneficial effect on insulin sensitivity, which may help control diabetes as explained earlier.

Soluble fibres can also help lower LDL ("bad") blood cholesterol by interfering with the absorption of dietary cholesterol.[1]

Sources of soluble fibre: lentils, apples, oranges, pears, oat bran, strawberries, nuts, flaxseeds, beans, dried peas, blueberries, psyllium, cucumbers, celery, carrots, porridge (oatmeal) & oat cereal.

Insoluble fibre is considered gut healthy, because it has a laxative effect & adds bulk to your diet, helping prevent constipation.

These fibres do not dissolve in water, so they pass through the gastrointestinal tract relatively intact & speed up the passage of food & waste. Insoluble fibers are mainly found in whole grains & vegetables.

---

1 http://www.ncbi.nlm.nih.gov/pubmed/25346913

Sources of insoluble fibre: seeds, nuts, barley, couscous, brown rice, bulgur, zucchini, celery, broccoli, cabbage, onions, tomatoes, carrots, cucumbers, green beans, dark leafy vegetables, raisins, grapes, fruit, root-vegetable skins, whole wheat, whole grains, wheat bran, corn bran,

Both types of fibre are found as natural elements in plants, fruit, vegetables & grains. They're another good reason to eat fresh organic real food in comparison to processed man-made food alternatives.

Consuming a combination of both soluble & insoluble fibre is ideal.

A balanced diet will take care of that, or you can simply supplement it. We'll talk more about this later.

So why do we need it?

Having sufficient fibre in your diet helps create bulk in your digestive tract. It actually bulks up around your other digested food & moves the stool, plus any harmful carcinogens, through your body at a faster rate.

This is a good reason to get enough fibre, especially if the rest of your diet is not healthy.

When you don't have enough fibre in your diet, you know all about it. You become constipated - sluggish & bloated.

Having a clean & healthy colon is another key to optimal health & fitness, which is why I'm a big fan of getting enough fibre in your diet.

Fibre also helps you feel less hungry, but because it's not actually absorbed, it aids in fat loss & controlling your eating habits in a number of positive ways.

One of those ways is to slow the release of the energy from carbs into your blood stream. So for instance, if you have not mastered cutting out the sugary stuff yet, making sure you have adequate fiber coming into your system will manage the rate at which the sugar hits your bloodstream (a good thing).

When you manage this process as described above your body is less stressed, as your blood sugar level is more consistent & you do not have to produce as much Insulin (another good thing).

It's a simple way to improve your diet by adding something rather than just restricting certain foods – as I talked about earlier. As you gain the benefits of this you can then improve your food choice, which is the next step on your road to even greater success with your body & career.

Principle Exercise 17
Increase Fibre

This is extremely beneficial for four main reasons:

1) *It slows down glucose & insulin response to your meals, helping balance your blood-sugar level.*

2) *It provides detoxification.*

3) *It gives you a feeling of fullness (satiety).*

4) *It protects the mucosa of your colon.*

Healthy gut = healthy immune system = strong body & brain.

Pick up a fibre supplement from your local health shop or order one online, you can visit my website for this.

Consume thirty grams of fibre per day split in two doses:

Fifteen grams in the morning (approximately one heaped tablespoon) & fifteen grams in the evening, after your last meal is good.

Dissolve the powder into a small glass of clean water, mix it & drink.

Principle 17
I Maintain A Healthy Bowel

A healthy bowel promotes a healthy immune system, which stimulates a healthy mind.

Remember that there are two kinds of fibre: soluble & insoluble.

Soluble fiber dissolves into a gel in water & helps control glucose levels & blood sugar. Insoluble fiber absorbs water & adds bulk to your digestive tract, which moves food through your digestive system.

Add fibre to your daily diet You will find it easier to control your body fat.

Reduce your risk to diseases like cancer, diabetes & heart disease.

About eighteen to thirty grams a day keeps bowel movements flowing optimally.

Achieve this by eating a selection of the foods listed, & I always recommend supplementing fibre.

If supplementing, put a heaped tablespoon in a little water in the morning & drink. Repeat this in the evening

Adding an extra tablespoon at lunch won't hurt.

When you improve the health of your gut you will notice that you feel stronger in body & mind. You will boost your immune system & not fall ill as often. Your mind will be able to focus with ease & your skin will become clearer.

These are just a few benefits. This is a critical skill to master on your road to Optimal Health & Fitness.

The Big Benefits of Low GI

A recent Harvard study proved that low glycemic-index (GI) foods are better at maintaining metabolism during fat loss & promoting cardiovascular health.[1,2]

A low-GI food releases its energy into your bloodstream slower than a high-GI food will.

This gives you better control over blood sugar & insulin production. When you eat low GI foods the rate at which your body has to respond to your meal is slower & therefore less stressful on your system.

If there is a quick rise in blood sugar, your body is alerted & rushed through insulin production, with the aim of rebalancing your blood-sugar level.

If this happens regularly, certain areas of your body become resistant to insulin (receptor sites). Then you need to make even more insulin to balance your blood sugar, as your body cannot receive the appropriate amounts effectively, which increases internal stress through your system.

On the other hand, if your blood sugar rises slowly, your body responds accordingly & makes smaller amounts of insulin, as required.

The less insulin you make & the more sensitive you are to it, the easier it is for your body to maintain equilibrium.

Over production of insulin damages & ages your cells[3] Clearly the less damage to your cells the better.

---

1 http://www.ncbi.nlm.nih.gov/pubmed/17344493

2 http://www.hsph.harvard.edu/nutritionsource/carbohydrates/carbohydrates-and-blood-sugar/

3 http://www.sciencedaily.com/releases/2007/07/070719141139.htm

When you manage your energy levels, one effective way is to manage your blood sugar level, the quicker you positively respond to exercise, the healthier & more vital you are, the less exposed you are to disease & you will live longer.

Diabetics & Athletics

David Mendosa once said:

> When you make use of the glycemic index to prepare healthy meals, it helps to keep your blood glucose levels under control. This is especially important for people with diabetes, although athletes & people who are overweight also stand to benefit from knowing about this relatively new concept in good nutrition.

In the most part sticking to low-GI foods will eliminate processed, refined carbohydrates & baked or fried goods that simply poison your body.

If you still eat these types of food then it is time to stop. They reduce your potential, make you susceptible to toxins by damaging your digestive system & in turn your immune system.

At worst, set yourself a rule that you'll only eat these types of food a maximum of once a week, or on Sunday, straight after a healthy Sunday lunch.

We'll go over a little more theory & then we'll look at a food chart so you know you're always making a smart carbohydrate choice for each meal based on the GI options.

A Side Note

- Open your fridge. Likely, your water, meat & veggies are all in plastic containers or wrapped in plastic. A lot of these plastics contain Bisphenol A (BPA) &

other phthalates that are poisonous & leach into your food. Make sure your containers are BPA free.

- In the United States, a study by the Centers for Disease Control & Prevention found that 93 percent of urine samples taken from a random group of 2,517 people contained BPA.

Packaged, processed food is simply not good for you.

Your goal is to get your hands on whole, organic, fresh food on a daily basis.

Take thirty minutes to source your local farmers' market or your organic produce options, or have your assistant do it for you.

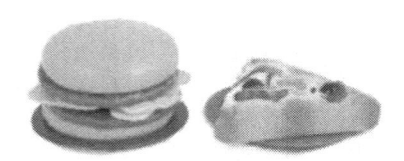

Once you've eaten fresh organic food for a couple of weeks you'll not only see & feel the difference, you'll taste it as well.

After eating organic produce for a while, when you come to eat a packaged or processed food you will taste the plastic or 'off taste' & not want to continue eating it. It's there, contributing to obesity & ill health. If you're eating it then it's holding you back from even greater success, vitality & optimal health.

It's time to lose plastic food from your diet—fast. Then watch your health improve—fast.

Is Your Bowel Healthy?

You must have heard that if you look through a person's trash, you can tell a lot about that person's lifestyle. The same goes for your bowel movements.

Do you monitor your bowel movements? You can tell a lot about what is happening with your health just by checking out what your body throws away every day.

The goal is to go to the bathroom several times a day—three is optimum—with no signs of constipation or diarrhea. You shouldn't have to push or strain to have a bowel movement.

Once you cut out higher-GI foods, junk food, fast food, packaged, processed food & sugar items, you'll quickly see an improvement in your bowel activity. Your bowel movements will become more regular & you'll pass your stools with no strain or discomfort.

I know this is a crap thing to talk about (excuse the pun) but it's worth the conversation.

If the described process is not your current experience then this must be addressed. The information I have been providing you & the preceding info will help to optimalise your experience & improve your overall health.

As a general rule

- Stool that appears white, clay-colored, black/tarry, ribbon-like, hard, or liquid is considered abnormal. If it persists for longer than three weeks, go see your doctor. This could be a sign of severe dehydration or an inability to absorb certain nutrients.

- A good healthy stool is easy to pass, will come on suddenly & spontaneously & is brown, soft & well formed.

- You can take immediate steps to improve on less-than-perfect stools. Remember that your stool is a response to your diet. Correct your diet & you'll correct your stool. You'll also improve the health of your bowel (which decreases your risk to cancers & keeps your immune system strong), alongside losing fat & having more energy.

Monitoring your bowel is about checking that your body is getting what it needs. If things are not flowing, eat more fibre & drink more water.

If your stool is too loose, eat more protein, consume more insoluble fibre, or supplement it two to three times a day as explained earlier.

Also think about what could have irritated your bowel. Often it's gluten (one in one hundred people are intolerant) that causes poor intestinal function.

Cereal Killer…

Like many hardworking individuals, you probably eat high-fibre cereal to stay regular. You'll have to switch from this, as many of these cereals contain high-fructose corn syrup & sugar & are generally high in carbs, with a very high GI.

One study from Michigan University found that with a well-known cereal brand, the box contained more nutrients than the food[1]

Eighteen rats were divided into three groups. One group were fed the cereal with water, the second group were fed the box that the cereal came in & water, the third group were fed rat chow & water.

The rats receiving the box became lethargic & eventually died of malnutrition. But the rats receiving cornflakes & water died before the rats that were given the box.

---

1 file:///Users/danielgrant/Downloads/NOC_Extruder.pdf

The last cornflake rat died on the day the first box rat died. Before death the cornflake rats developed schizophrenic behavior, threw fits, bit each other & finally went into convulsions.

Autopsy revealed dysfunction of the pancreas, liver and kidneys & degeneration of the nerves in the spine – all signs of "insulin shock."

This study suggests that there is more nourishment in the box that cold breakfast cereals come in than in the cereals themselves.

Millions of children & busy adults begin their day with a bowl of breakfast cereal thinking that it is healthy.

Could the toxic protein fragments in these cereals explain why so many of our children cannot concentrate at school? Or why more & more people these days are suffering from nutritional deficiencies, diabetes & nutritional dysfunction.[2]

This brings another meaning to the term cereal killer!

Since 1996 the number of people with diabetes has increased from 1.4 to 2.9 million people. By 2015 it is estimated that five million people will have diabetes. I'd suggest that what you choose to eat for breakfast has a dramatic affect over your long-term health.

This is a great example of the displacement foods I introduced you to earlier. These foods take more from your body as they are being digested than they provide you in nutrition.

This process slowly drains your health bank account until you are diseased, sick & taking lots of medication to keep you functioning… until you eventually die.

---

2 http://www.diabetes.org.uk/About_us/What-we-say/Statistics/Diabetes-in-the-UK-2013-Key-statistics-on-diabetes/

Get yourself back to "regular" by eating a healthy fresh food diet, raw sources of fibre or by taking a well-made dietary fibre supplement. I offer a few options of good fiber supplements through my website. Alternatively your local health shop should be able to guide you.

Chapter 11:
Your Nutritional Recovery

The doctor of the future will no longer treat the human frame with drugs, but rather will cure and prevent disease with nutrition.

—*Thomas Edison*

Recovering from the damage that the modern diet has done to your body will not be an easy task. It's not as simple as losing weight or eating right for a couple of days.

This chapter will walk you through the reasons why nutritional recovery needs to be a big part of your life.

As you begin to fix your diet, you'll notice that your body starts to reshape itself.

You have always had the power to heal & sculpt your body, but it only works if you manage your lifestyle, exercise, nutrition & supplementation effectively—which is what this book & my idea of 'Optimalism' are all about.

The Dangers of Carb Overuse

One effective way to quickly increase your overall level of health & fitness is to adopt a high-protein, low-carb diet. To reach a goal of losing fat & building quality muscle there must be an element of this type of diet involved for periods of time. This requires protein & lots of nutrients from certain vegetables with a sprinkle of fruit.

You will also require adequate amounts of amino acids & varying amounts of certain carbohydrates at specific points in your day.

The detail you can get into regarding this point is mind-boggling! It requires a book of its own, or several in fact. So here are some brief rules & a solid overview so you can start making smart, effective choices right away.

Blood Sugar Spikes…

When you eat a lot of carbohydrate-based foods that are processed & high GI, your blood-sugar levels spike & they often behave erratically for periods of time. This results in decreased metabolic function (the processes necessary for a living organism to survive) & fat gain.

Eating in this way will lead a person to insulin desensitisation. This is basically what happens with people who have type 2 diabetes, which can vary greatly in severity.

The term used to describe this is *insulin resistant. This is* predominantly caused by an unbalanced diet & the overconsumption of high-GI foods.

It basically means that your cells are becoming resistant to Insulin. It's the same as building up a tolerance for any substance, for instance alcohol or a drug, where you require more & more of the substance, over time, to have the same effect.

If you have previously struggled to experience results from your training routines no matter how hard & how much you train, then this is the first place to start looking for the answers.

If your diet is not tailored in a specific way - determined by your current physical status, then you might encourage fat gain, rather than muscle gain no matter how hard & often you train.

The more insulin-*resistant* you are, the more fat you'll put on when you eat high-carb foods & a high volume of carbs in relation to protein & 'good fat' (I'll explain these later). This process is highly stressful to your body, which means more fat gain around the middle.

If, however, you don't abuse yourself, but instead maintained a steady blood-sugar level, you could well be carb-tolerant. If you are already applying *Principle 14 of Optimalism* then you are on the right track.

If you also train a few times a week or at least keep yourself physically active, then you will benefit from a specific amount of carbohydrate intake.

Those who are lean & physically active, you may be one, may actually *deserve carbs* & it would be beneficial for you to consume some. Again the amount is dependent on a few specific variables.

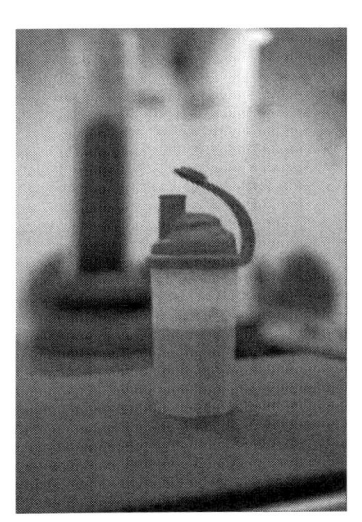

Your body needs to release energy efficiently when you exercise & use whatever protein foods you eat to build additional muscle.

This is why body builders often drink protein shakes. They help to bolster protein intake & are a bio-available (easily used by the body).

Your body quickly uses protein (whey protein is common in protein shakes) & amino acids in periods of "rest" after weight training, to heal torn muscle fibers & make them stronger & bigger.

That is one process required to take muscles from weak to strong & small to big, using nutrition.

How A Carb Habit Can Cause Disease

Eating a lot of carbohydrates may work for some people but not for most.

Carbohydrate intolerance is the inability to process the nutrient carbohydrate into a source of energy. These carbohydrates are predominantly sugars & starches. Lactose intolerance, the sugar found in milk, is widespread & affects up to 70% of the worlds population.[1]

That means there is a seventy five percent chance that you are carb intolerant. Keep in mind that there is also a twenty five percent chance that you are *carb tolerant*. How can you determine if you are carb tolerant?

A very good way due to its un-invasive approach is by using a BioSignature assessment.[2] This is a body fat test using calipers (metal pinchers with a dial) which also provides a feedback about your hormonal profile.

According to this system you can determine if a person is eating too much carbs than what they actually need. Certain areas of your body contain receptor sites for hormones. Simply put, where you lay down fat provides a feedback of what is going on with the related hormone.

With this system, you can achieve 98 percent accuracy in body-fat testing.

---

1 http://medical-dictionary.thefreedictionary.com/carbohydrate+intolerance

2 http://www.poliquingroup.com/upload/content/biosigtext_pracuse.pdf

The reason I suggest testing your body fat regularly is that what you eat results in what you look like. Obvious, right? But the nuts & bolts of it is that the specific receptor sites located at specific positions throughout your body tell a story about your health.

As these sites shift, for better or worse, you get a reading of what your diet & lifestyle are doing for your physique & performance.

Getting your body-fat percentage tested regularly allows you to see the changes as they happen, from when you cut out carbs completely, to when you reintegrate them.

Your Carb Situation

Ignoring this is a great way to ensure that you remain unhealthy forever. Choosing to avoid high-carb foods for periods of time gives your body the chance to heal. Test it & see.

Not all carbs are made equal!

Unfortunately for some, most carbohydrates contribute to a highly inflammatory condition inside their body, which is the perfect climate for disease.

This is especially true for age-related diseases. There is nothing normal about getting a disease when you get older, it may be common but it is not normal. Eliminating specific carbs can dramatically reduce your risk & in a lot of cases prevent disease.

Some 80 percent of your local supermarket is dedicated to selling carbohydrates. You never stood a chance. Most think that fat is the bad guy. Which has some element of truth, particularly when you consider the quality of the fat – think avocado compared to cheap deep-frying fat.

Alternatively, here's how carbs cause disease in your body:

- *Signs of what is being called "Excessive Carbohydrate Consumption Syndrome"* appear as body fat increases: diabetes, heart disease, cancer, gallbladder disease, degenerative bone diseases, the related list of issues could on.

- *Certain carbohydrates can damage your intestinal tract* causing leaky gut syndrome, irritable bowel syndrome (IBS) & autoimmune diseases. The sugar in these carbs also damages arteries & blood vessels, which can lead to heart attack, stroke & heart disease if it continues over time.

Think about the average person's day (maybe your average day?): cereal for breakfast, sandwiches for lunch, or rolls, pies, bagels, or muffins. Then onto dinner for pasta, rice, or starchy tacos—*carb overload.*

A study conducted by the Center for Disease Control (CDC) in the United States highlighted that over fifty percent of daily energy was coming from carbohydrates. Bear in mind that the US has rising obesity rates. Could excessive refined carbohydrate intake be part of the problem?[1]

Instead of your High-Carb Breakfasts

- Don't eat anything. Train instead. *Then* eat your high-protein meal, adding mushrooms, onions, tomatoes, or even green vegetables after your workout.

- Some advocate this style of fasting while training & some do not. Test it for yourself. The first couple of times you try this method, you may feel strange, but your body will adapt quickly.

---

1 http://www.cdc.gov/nchs/data/nhanes/databriefs/calories.pdf

- Some report they can train much more intensely on an empty stomach, while others report they run out of energy. Depending on your goal & level of health, test out alternative methods from time to time. I will provide you with some structure around this later.

- Mix eggs with spinach, tomatoes, onion & mushrooms to make a vegetable omelette. They all contain good protein levels, even though they aren't meats. Eat this with a protein of your choice.

- If you really want to feel alert & energised, eat meat & nuts for breakfast. I got this tip from Charles Poliquin, as it's one of his trademarks. Think steak & cashew nuts, or lamb chops & pistachios. The combination is up to you.

- This will boost dopamine levels (your neurotransmitter for concentration & focus), making your mind sharper & also leave you feeling fuller for longer through a slower release of energy into your bloodstream—to name only a few positives.

Dealing with Sugar & Carb Cravings

When you cut down or stop eating carbohydrates & sugar, guess what? You have withdrawal. Some researchers say it's as addictive as cocaine [2]

The high-GI, high-fat combo causes similar reactions within our brains.

No wonder so many people struggle to cut these foods out of their diet. Sugar is a drug! If you learn to manage your food intake

---

2 http://www.conncoll.edu/news/news-archive/2013/student-faculty-research-suggests-oreos-can-be-compared-to-drugs-of-abuse-in-lab-rats.htm#.VI6iZqSsX_Y

effectively, you'll suffer fewer cravings & achieve more positive results with your health & fitness.

Cortisol (stress hormone) & Insulin (sugar management hormone) have an inverse relationship. When your stress levels are high, your cortisol rises. You crave sugar to give you energy to get through the stressful event & lower your Cortisol levels.

As you consume the sugar, your insulin levels rise. As insulin rises your cortisol levels are subdued. Voilà—you feel less stressed.

This is one reason you crave sugar & carbs when you are stressed.

Eating ice cream, for example, floods your body with sugar. Insulin levels rise & the cortisol recedes. That's why you feel satisfied & happier once you've eaten something sweet or full of carbs. But remember— all carbohydrates are not made equal.

There are lots of better alternatives that you can eat with relative security, as long as you eat them in moderation & they do not become the center of your diet again.

Here are some things you need to know about sugar & carb cravings:

- It's OK to feel hungry. Hunger is not bad. You can view hunger as your body burning fat. As long as you consume the recommended calorie intake (Approx. 2000 for men & 1500 for women) from nutritious foods each day you will be fine. Feeling hunger for a portion of each day, between dinner & breakfast for example, is not such a bad thing. Besides, going hungry is better for you than eating a *chemical-sugar pie.*

- You should aim to be hungry for a period of time each day, as it will promote the use of stored fat & efficient nutrient uptake when you eat—as long as that meal is high in nutrients & not just empty calories. The period of time you feel hungry for can be fluctuated – for instance in may range from eight to sixteen hours. More about this later.

- Drink at least two to three liters of water every day. Most of the population is in a permanent state of dehydration & this can cause you to feel hungry, when, in fact, you're just thirsty.

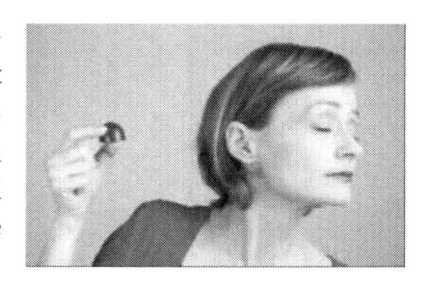

- As a rule, don't drink anything with sugar or imitation sugar in it. Instead, stick to clear teas, coffee, nondairy drinks & of course water.

If you are serious about achieving optimal health & fitness, then you must live through any carbohydrate & sugar withdrawal for a short period of time.

You may feel uncomfortable, have cravings & even experience nausea, but it will subside considerably within a few days & disappear completely after one to two weeks.

Fat Loss Made Easy

Fat loss can be made a lot easier when you manage your carb intake. In fact, just by substituting simple, high-processed carbs with more natural real-food carbs like green vegetables, salads & a little fruit, you'll flood your body with nutrients that also help burn fat rather store fat

You get a positive double whammy. Keep in mind that for your body to respond at its best to weight training, you must eat lots of protein & apply carbs at specific times throughout your day.

For fat loss without much concern for bodybuilding, you can reduce your carbs to a minimum & then slowly reintegrate certain ones as your tolerance improves once more.

You can reposition yourself as carb tolerant if you give yourself a break from carbs for a period of time. In most cases, your pancreas & most of your body, will view this as a welcome rest.

You can find lists of healthy carb food choices anywhere online & we'll go through some later in the book.

The goal of course is to own your body shape, so you can perform & look your best all the time.

It can be a trying process, with toxins leaving your body as the fat melts away, but it could be the single most rewarding thing you'll ever achieve in your life, which promotes success in every other area of your life.

Fat Loss, Short-term Fasting & Blood Chemistry

When you stretch your meal gaps, a form of fasting, your body burns fat. It's a total myth that this is bad for you. In fact, you can use this to great effect as long as you compensate the feeling of hunger with your next meal, your calorie intake is sufficient every day, you eat highly nutritious food & supplement according to your specific requirements.

If you want to lose fat quickly, I can introduce you to an approach using your meal gaps to stimulate better health & better aesthetics.

For instance, instead of eating breakfast at seven o'clock, have a big lunch at eleven. I teach this approach to clients & those who participate in my 7Week-Body-Transformation course.

Your insulin levels will stay low up to that first meal. The training that you may do in the morning will tap into your energy stores & you will become a fat-burning machine.

Your body does best when you keep it guessing. Change your eating habits from time to time. Alter your food choices. Switch your training style.

All the consistently changing variables will stimulate greater health if they are based on science.

Many studies show that structured, scientific fasting improves your blood chemistry[1] Blood pressure, blood fats, cholesterol/triglycerides & insulin levels can all be improved by an appropriate use of fasting techniques[2] Dr Michael Mosley has created one system around this concept called the fast diet.

You must, of course, do this in combination with a healthy diet, good exercise plan & appropriate supplementation if you want the fastest, safest & longest-lasting results.

Be aware if you have kidney or liver issues, you will need to be careful taking this approach, make sure to consult with your health care professional or doctor.

Select Your Diet Plan

You must have noticed how many diet options are available. If there was one diet that worked for everyone all of the time, someone would have discovered it by now.

The truth is that one way of eating is not the *Holy Grail*. Just like regular changes to your training stimulus in order to keep growing muscle & improve sporting performance are the keys to success, you also require regular changes to your diet.

---

1 http://www.ncbi.nlm.nih.gov/pubmed/25458830

2 http://thefastdiet.co.uk/why-fast/

This may come in the form of food selection, from high to moderate protein, moderate to high fat & low to moderate—& at certain time even high carb.

This variant can also be applied to meal gaps, or the amount of time between meals. This concept has been coined "intermittent fasting."

Although I don't advocate eating this way 100 percent of the time, I've seen massive improvements in people's body composition & level of health through applying this system.

It basically involves fasting for a period of your day. For instance, you eat dinner at eight o'clock. Usually, you'll end your fast by breaking it at around six thirty—this is appropriately named '*breakfast*' or *break fast*.

This fast lasted ten-and-a-half hours. This period of time can change from day to day depending on your lifestyle. So, what intermittent fasting does is expands the period of time between your last meal & your first meal the next day.

Twenty-Four-Hour Cavemart

If you think back to caveman times, there wasn't access to twenty-four-hour supermarkets & our caveman ancestors went hungry on occasions.

Granted, they only lived to about thirty-five, on average, but they didn't suffer with souring obesity rates either.

Perhaps with the choices we have & our knowledge of the past, we can achieve balance between health, function, high performance & longevity.

So what you do with intermittent fasting (IF) is stretch the period between dinner & breakfast. For example, you eat dinner at eight o'clock.

The next solid food you put in your mouth will not be until eight in the morning.

As most people don't eat through the night while they are sleeping (sleep eaters1) then most people's meal gap between dinner & breakfast is usually six to eight hours.

What IF (Intermittent Fasting) does is stretch that period of time to twelve, fourteen, sixteen & in some cases, eighteen hours.

I suggest starting small & building up in half-hour increments every two days until you reach your maximum fasting time. A common intermittent fast split is sixteen – eight. This is sixteen hours of fasting followed by an eight-hour eating window.

So you'll do all your eating within that eight-hours. For example between, midday & eight o'clock. Fast from eight o'clock to midday & repeat.

It's important that you consume an appropriate amount of calories within your eating window. Constantly under-eating only leads to binging, bad food choices, vitamin & mineral deficiencies & eventually illness.

Intermittent fasting also gives you the benefits of saving time. Breakfast is commonly skipped & a large brunch can be eaten in its place a few hours later.

It can also be integrated however it suits you. This way, you can eat large breakfasts if you prefer them, & eat dinner earlier – several hours before bed.

If you also like eating till you're full, then eat a large dinner as well. It all depends on how you prefer to experience each meal. A little experimentation with these techniques will determine what is the right system for you.

Principle Exercise 18
Fast Time

Some simple rules for your IF plan:

• *Keep in mind that you can complete the bulk of your fasting at night. This way, you're asleep & don't experience hunger while you're trying to work. Start your fast one to two hours before bed & continue it for two or more hours after waking.*

• *Once you start eating (break your fast) then eat regularly throughout the day. Triggering your hunger response will help streamline your metabolism & accelerate your fat-burning power. After you break your fast, aim to eat every one & a half to two hours.*

• *Having to time your meals helps you plan better. You'll look ahead & plan what you'll eat—make sure this is a healthy choice. I'll help you understand what a healthy choice is throughout this book.*

• *Start the length of your first fast for twelve hours.*

• *Keep this time for at least two days or up to one week to allow yourself to get used to the pattern & feeling of the fast.*

If after the settling in period you feel fine with this period of fast, increase it by one hour. Hold that time for at least two days to one week then increase by one hour again if all is going well.

• *Keep this process going until you reach a sixteen hour fast. You will have then reached a sixteen-eight intermittent fasting pattern.*

• *Use this for a period of two to four weeks then return back to having breakfast or a meal gap of no more than eight hours.*

Principle 18

I Intermittently Fast For Optimal Health & Performance

By applying this technique, you can stimulate greater fat loss, improve your blood fat levels, improve fasting insulin (useful to determine insulin resistance) & improve cholesterol status.[1]

You will also, in the process, learn greater control—physical & mental—improve your meal-planning skills & understand exactly what your body needs to be at optimum.

Through this technique you can master your body fat & health status.

This is a skill that can be honed; once you've honed it, you won't look back, as you'll be mastering your body shape & health for life.

A major benefit from IF is that you rest your digestive tract. Most people would benefit massively by giving their digestive system a little rest & allowing it to heal. Followed by high nutrient meals that do not contain any food intolerances or allergies.

This is a system to use intermittently. You can have dramatic effect on your health & body fat by applying it in an appropriate way as I have outlined for you.

It is another tool in your armory. Use it wisely on your path to your personal best.

---

1 http://www.sciencedaily.com/releases/2011/04/110403090259.htm

Working with Portion Control

Portion sizes matter—just ask McDonald's. They quickly realised that if they made larger amounts of food available at cheaper prices, people would always choose the larger amount. It's simple—you're getting more for your money.

But is this a healthy way to make your food choices?

If you're going to sort out your nutrition, then you need to sort out your portion sizes. Too many people in the Western world eat too much.

Not only do people eat too much, but they eat too much of the wrong type of food—meaning low nutrition.

This causes cravings for more food soon after finishing a meal even though they have eaten a large sized meal.

Why is it the wrong type of food? The simple answer is this—raise your hand now if you want to increase your body fat over the next two weeks.

I'll bet you didn't raise your hand. In most cases, eating a certain type of food guarantees that you'll gain fat. Eat the right types of food & you can guarantee the opposite.

- The majority of English men—65 percent—are overweight[2] We have a culture of eating more than we need, because we are used to eating solely for taste—& food that isn't so good for us is created to appeal to our taste buds.

According to the National Health Service in the UK (NHS) the amount of food you eat should depend on your size & physical activity level. Eating the right number of calories is the key. A calorie is a unit

---

1 http://vizhub.healthdata.org/obesity/

of energy found in food. The more calories food has, the more energy you absorb into your body.

If your body doesn't use all this energy, it stores it as fat. That's why when you gain weight, you've eaten more calories than what you burnt in a twenty-four-hour period.

One mainstream theory of how to burn fat is to reduce your calorie intake while exercising. By doing this you create a calorie deficit where you burn up stored fat as fuel Simple—or maybe not so simple.

- According to the NHS Men need approximately 2,500 calories a day to *maintain* healthy body weight & women require approximately 2000 calories[3]

- Remember I coach a different calorie intake to this in order to stimulate changes in body composition as described earlier.

Get used to the idea that food contains energy & consuming too much energy is not good for you when done consistently for prolonged periods of time. Consciously select your portion sizes. Principles 14, 15, 16 & 17 within this book help you structure that choice for each meal.

Eating meals that contain lots of green vegetables can help to replace the stodge food that so many people are used to.

Eating more green vegetables has four main positives:

1) They are low in calories, but fill you up.
2) They are low GI (have a slow effect on blood sugar), so you can eat as much as you like of these types of food. You will feel fuller after each meal as you have simply eaten more.

3 http://www.nhs.uk/chq/pages/1126.aspx?categoryid=51

3) Green vegetables are high in fiber, which helps
   maintain your blood sugar & promotes a healthy bowel.
4) Green vegetables—the fresher, the better—are
   loaded with vitamins & minerals.

Read labels. You need a good reason to put food in your mouth. Make sure that it is organic, nutritious & that it adds up to a reasonable calorie threshold as outlined.

Cut Outs & Food Increases

You are what you eat. Have you ever heard that? It is quite literally true. Your body rebuilds itself from the nutrients you supply it with.

If, like many others, you have been consistently eating carbs & sugar, then you are most likely overweight, exhausted & ill—or at least well on your way to this situation.

Do you have to fuel yourself with coffee or sports drinks (caffeine) all day long in order to have the energy to make it through the day?

To perform at your best, you have to eat a healthy, balanced diet. You should be getting a solid idea of what that consists of.

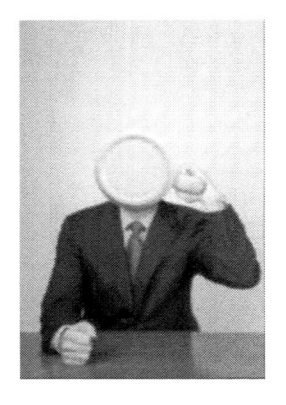

Each & every food choice you make affects your body on a cellular & hormonal level.

The nutritional content of your food goes into creating your cell membranes, bone marrow, blood, hormones, your eyes—everything. You are created from the food you eat.

So think about what you've eaten in the past twenty-four hours. Will your next eyeball have telescopic focus, or could you end up blind as a bat?

If your answer is the latter, then you need to cut out the bad foods & increase the good ones.

Immediate Steps to Take

- *Cut out sugary soft drinks & energy drinks*—any drink that is high-calorie, energy drinks, full of fat, sugar, or milk (dairy).

- *Only drink tea, coffee & water* (herbals or your normal blend), coffee (in moderation & at the ideal times of day) & water. A little alcohol will probably not kill you, but it also wouldn't do you any harm to go without for a week or two. Could you manage that? This will reduce one form of stress load on your system giving it time to heal & be at more of an optimal state.

- *Only eat organic food.* While organic food is not always available, organic fruits & vegetables are packed with the nutrients you need. Arguably more important is that they are also lower in chemical residues, which poison your body from the inside out.

- *Only eat free-range, naturally reared meats.* Avoid all battery-cage farms, fish farms & canned meats. They will cause dysfunction within your body if eaten consistently over periods of time.

- *Do not eat sugar or high-fructose corn syrup,* artificial sweeteners (aside from stevia) & eat high-GI carbs sparingly. They will kill you slowly. Stevia, once outlawed due to it being an unknown quantity has been used for years in South America. Studies now show that it can help to lower hypertension (high blood pressure) & hyperglycemia (high blood glucose)[1] It now equates for 40% of the sweetener market in Japan.

- *Add lots of fresh vegetables to your menu.* There are literally dozens you have probably never even tasted. Some can be cooked to taste absolutely incredible.

- *Drink clean/filtered water,* along with lots of herbal-infused waters or teas for natural health promotion. These natural herbs all have their own health promoting qualities. Don't miss out on them.

Before you put that next bite of donut into your body, consider that the greasy, sugary disease-causing carb bomb will be all your body has to fix itself for the next several hours.

You & your body deserve better than that.

If you expect the best from your body & brain then fuel yourself in an optimal way.

---

1 http://www.ncbi.nlm.nih.gov/pubmed/20370653

Chapter 12:
Rules for Food Recovery

We may find in the long run that tinned food is a deadlier weapon than the machine-gun.

—George Orwell

In this final section on nutrition, I want to remind you of something important. It doesn't matter how badly you've eaten up till now.

The human body can & will recover if you consistently & conscientiously give it the right foods at the right time.

There are rules involved in food recovery & it will take some getting used to. Moving from a high-carb diet to living a relatively carb-free or low-carb lifestyle is a challenge.

However, you have the willpower & drive to succeed when you put your mind to it. You show it in your career & in the rest of your life.

It's time for that focus to appear in this area of your life—from right now.

Your Food Choices Matter

Imagine if a breaking-news story came across the television right now: "What You Eat Directly Affects Your Short-Term Health."

People would panic. Of course, many studies exist proving that food affects us this way, but because we tend to only experience the long-term effects, there are always "ifs" & "buts" about food & how it affects us in the short-term.

So let me seize this opportunity to emphasise what you are already aware of: most of the food in most people's immediate reach is pure rubbish.

Supermarket food may not be your wisest choice due to the lack of freshness & low nutrient value. Depending on which restaurant you choose to eat in will have a massive bearing on your health – particularly if you eat there regularly.

It's a pity that this is the case, but when profit is involved, motives no longer remain as simple as "good health." Instead the cheapest works best. Foods that last the longest on the shelves all take precedence over healthy counterparts.

- Eating well is not a short-term commitment. It's a lifelong commitment. What you eat now will affect you tomorrow & in the years to come.

- *Simple, nutritious food that human beings have been eating for thousands of years is the best kind of food.*

- If it's safe to eat it raw & your gut health is good, then do so.

- The longer you eat healthy food, the higher performance levels you will be able to reach. You'll develop leaner, stronger muscles; better skin; & you'll look younger for longer—& live a longer happier life.

The Food-as-Fuel Theory

Food should be used as the medicine of the human body. A calorie is a unit of energy & so, food should be seen as fuel.

You may need to shift your relationship with food that goes beyond a messy, dependent, emotional relationship. Just because something tastes good does not mean it is good for you. That much is obvious.

The problem is that for too long, most people made their meal choices from pure taste, rather than from taste & health. Are you one of these people?

You can use food & the fluid you drink to facilitate increased performance in your workouts, work life, social & personal life—or the direct opposite.

Food should inject energy into your body & mind, which can then be spent on healthy & happy pursuits.

Quick Application:

- Plan your meals ahead of time. When dinner is being prepared, have twice as much made. This will do you for lunch or breakfast the next day. Plan this yourself or with the person who prepares most of your meals.

- Have direct input into the quality & quantity of food your meals are made from. Eat as many meals as possible from a choice of the best quality produce that money can buy. This is the smartest investment you can make – *fact.*

- You can get your day's meals delivered to your home or office. Source & confirm a meal provider. There are plenty of options to choose from these days. Which is a reputable company with the highest quality produce? Choose the best.

- As mentioned earlier, to achieve & remain at optimal health & fitness you will need to alter your patterns regularly. When you are not in a period of intermittent fasting, aim to eat one to two meals before you work out & eat again after your workout to fuel maximum muscle growth.

- Hydrate before & after working out to keep your body in peak condition.

- Aim to eat regularly throughout the day. Every two to three hours is good a good rule of thumb. When in a fasting phase, after you break the fast you should be eating regularly throughout the rest of your day until the eating window closes as described earlier.

- Hunger is nothing more than a signal from your brain & body that you require fuel - energy or nutrients. Make your selections specifically & in advance to enhance your health & your entire life will shift for the better.

- If you don't engage in heavy, long-distance cardio workouts—which I advise against—you will not need to devour high-carb foods that can be detrimental to most people's health & wellness. Instead, low GI foods, protein & smart fats will provide you with optimal energy & nutrients to achieve your personal best.

So you see, food is actually fuel.

The fact that it tastes good is an added bonus. In the old days (pre–Cooking Channel), we knew food was safe to eat if it tasted good. If it tasted bad, we would not eat it. We knew it was bad if it was old. Nowadays, these tastes, the age of the food & hidden poisons can be masked to taste & look good.

Principle Exercise 19
Fail to Prepare—Prepare to Fail

Quickly plan your eating times for the next day;

Each evening, take up to 5 minutes thinking about the following:

- **When is the best time(s) to eat throughout your day?**

When will you eat breakfast (fasting or not)
When is the next gap?
How long do you have to eat?
What food will you eat in that time – What food is available
How can you easily implement eating well throughout your day?

Have a brief outline of your eating times & plan
your meals for each day in advance.

This may seem extreme but with a schedule that is non-stop you
can easily lose track of your diet & in turn your body shape &
eventually your health.
Every meal has an affect on the homeostasis of your body (balance
of your internal systems) hormones, body fat, neurotransmitters,
energy levels etc.
A little pre-thought can go a very long way.

- **When is the best time(s) to train?**

Whenever possible plan your week of training times in advance,
spacing them appropriately within your day.
Pre-plan the night before when you will fit in your training.
This is important if you train alone, not so if you have a personal
trainer.

Principle 19
I Am Meticulous When Making Plans

Pre-plan your eating & training times into your schedule.

This can be as simple as a thought ahead of time.

You'll be surprised at how well this works for adherence to a specific eating plan as used in Principle 14: Eat For Optimal Health & Fitness

One healthy meal will not solve all of your health issues (if you have any) or create a fully functional body.

Just like one great workout will not deliver a toned muscular physique.

These things take time. It is the next 50+ meals & the next 50+ workouts that are going to make the difference to your health, fitness & performance levels.

The great thing is, the closer you remain to the path outlined the more vital you will feel each step of the way, the more intensely you will be able to focus for longer & longer periods of time, the more stress you will be able to handle as your body can recover optimally

Only then do you reach your Optimal state of being.
Only then do you experience your full potential.

It's time to shift your focus.

Follow the Principles of Optimalism as though your life depends on it
—because it really does.

A Word On Juicing

You would have likely heard about juicing or even been part of a juicing craze. These fads tend to bubble up from time to time like most things in the health & fitness industry.

Well I am here to tell you that juicing is one fad that you should keep participating in.

It consists of juicing (or blending) a bunch of green vegetables (or fruit) to make a smoothie or juice like drink.

In simple terms juicing is the equivalent of taking in a high dose of bioavailable (easily absorbed) vitamins & minerals. Think of it like taking a multivitamin but instead of a pill the nutrients are coming from real food.

I advocate supplementation simply because most people do not get enough nutrients in their system on a daily basis. They are obese & under nourished! Remember I talked you through this earlier.

So in my opinion supplements are good, essential for some people, however it is obvious that the more nutrients that you can obtain from real food the better this will be for you in the long run.

As I talked you through the dangers of over consumption of carbs you may be wondering about carbohydrate intake at this point?

The main thing to remember here is that green vegetables are so low on the GI scale that you could eat the entire green section of the grocery store without negatively affecting your body fat. In fact it would likely do you a world of good.

Problem being you'd struggle to eat that much food! So it's highly nutritious, filling & cheap – a very good combination I'm sure you agree?

This is where juicing comes in. You can juice a large plate piled high with green vegetables & that will make one large green juice that you can easily drink over a 5-10 minute period. It would take longer to eat that amount. Then you can do this two to three times each day.

Lastly, as talked about earlier be aware of the amount of fruit you consume. Yes fruit is good for you but the timing & amount is critical if you want to balance your blood sugar level throughout every day.

Remember not all fruits are made equal... & green veg will not spike your blood sugar – which is a good thing, most of the time.

The Key to Success

You likely have a hectic schedule, like most of my clients. That is why preparation is the key to success here. You can easily run out of food when reducing your carb intake is the goal.

Make sure you take the time to prepare for initial waves of hunger in the first two to three weeks. Precook lunches the night before. Boil eggs & keep fresh raw vegetables & fruits handy as snacks.

It may even suit you to keep some precooked lean protein to take with you during the day. This is to pre-vent you from giving into hunger & buying that pie or fast-food burger.

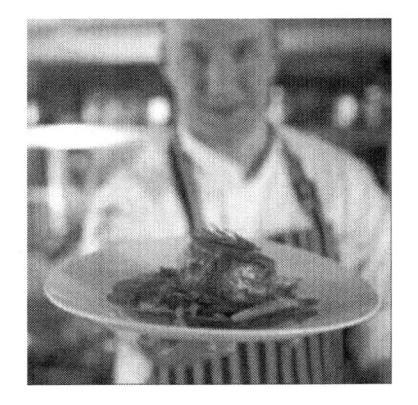

You don't have time to put poison in your body, not if you want to achieve an optimal state & remain at the top of your game.

That means always thinking ahead about your food & training schedules, just as you do with your work sched-ule. Live through Principle 18.

Precook meals, carry your own fresh water, use stevia instead of other sweeteners or sugar & stick to your healthy goals.

Or hire someone to do all of the prep for you. Either way, get it handled, starting today. Prepare the surroundings for your body & mind to reach & remain within an optimal state, just as your career has.

Perusing the Food Charts

What You Can & Should Eat

Be aware of any food intolerances you may have. I strongly suggest that you test for this. I use a simple blood test.

If undiagnosed, food intolerances can wreak havoc on your gut & your overall health, not to mention cause fat gain.

Ideally, rotate your foods & don't eat the same food every day for six months straight—this type of eating brings on intolerances.

Your Food Choices

Protein

Choose an appropriate amount, Principle 14 will determine this, of one of the following for every main meal:

- Chicken
- Turkey
- Beef (fillet is leanest, but you can vary your selection)
- Lamb
- Pork
- Venison

- Fish (variety—alternate through as many as possible)
- Prawns (quality is critical)

Snack

Optional: add to main meal, or *use as a* snack

- Bacon (organic, the leaner, the better)
- Quality ham (organic, the leaner, the better)
- Turkey rashers or cuts of organic turkey
- Eggs
- Smoked salmon
- A quality protein powder (highly advised to rotate your protein supplement)

Carbohydrates

Vegetables

Choose one or two for every main meal. As these food choices are low GI they will not affect your blood sugar in a negative way so feel free to use large amounts of them for each meal:

- **Asparagus**
- **Celery**
- **Green beans**
- **Cabbage**
- **Green leaves**
- **Lettuce**
- **Cucumber**
- **Broccoli**
- **Cauliflower**
- **Miracle noodles** (www.MiracleNoodle.com)
- **Miracle rice** (www.MiracleNoodle.com)
- **Spinach**

- **Brussels sprouts**
- **Mushrooms**
- **Onions**
- **Kidney beans**
- **Kale**
- **Mung beans**
- **Carrots (as slightly higher GI use more sparingly)**
- **Sweet potato (as higher GI use more sparingly – plan using Principle 14)**

Grains

- **Quinoa**

Fruit

One piece of fruit per day, eaten on its own as a snack.

When following Principle 14 you will be using the grams in weight to choose amounts of foods that you will be eating.

Or to help you judge portion size one large handful of smaller fruits for this example equals one piece.

- **Berries, All (Your first choice fruit: low GI, low calorie, high antioxidant, taste good. Google a full list & rotate your way through that list over weeks & months)**
- **Cherries**
- **Plum**
- **Apple**
- **Peach**
- **Tomatoes**

- Peppers
- Chili peppers

Fat

Attempt to only eat these fats. They are smart fats that promote enhanced brain activity & function of your cells.

- Virgin coconut oil
- Butter
- Extra-virgin olive oil
- Nuts (all, as long as you do not have allergies)
- Avocado

Dairy

- Milk (in moderation)
- Lactose-free milk (this is better if you have a lactose intolerance)
- Natural Greek yogurt (this should not be flavoured or sweetened & also be naturally zero fat)
- Cheese (to be used in moderation): cheddar, Babybel light cheese, Leerdammer cheese, quark, cottage cheese, feta, goat, sheep & so on. The quality of the cheese matters. The amount you eat is also critical.

Extra & Beverages

For use throughout certain parts of your day. Remember to be caffeine free from 4pm onwards – everyday.

- Tea
- Coffee

- **Water**
- **Stevia—a sweetener**

Herbs & Spices

- **Sea Salt**
- **Cinnamon**
- **Garlic**
- **Ginger**
- **Cayenne**
- **Turmeric**
- **Mint**
- **Basil**
- **Dill**
- **Sage**
- **Clove**
- **Fennel**
- **Oregano**
- **Rosemary**
- **Parsley**
- **Chives**
- **Thyme**
- **Chili (+flakes)**

Little Tips

- Do not eat processed meat or fish (like canned tuna).

- Do not eat foods containing wheat or gluten.

- Limit your potato, pasta, bread & rice intake for a period of time, until you are carb tolerant (sensitive to insulin) again.

- Make protein & vegetables the stars of your meals.

Principle Exercise 20
Create A One-Week Outline Of Your Meals

This should take no more than 30 minutes to complete.

Based on the food choice list on the previous pages, devise a meal plan that includes different varieties of food, focus on protein & vegetables.

As mentioned earlier food rotation is a good idea if you want to avoid food intolerances that lead to allergic reactions, allergies, illness, bloating, gas & a number of other conditions, which are actually avoidable.

This mostly applies to protein due to the more intricate digestive processes required to absorb & utilise the food. However it also applies to vegetables & fruit in that you should vary your sources of vitamins & minerals to ensure you get the full spectrum of nourishment on offer.

My goal is to help you achieve optimal health & fitness. Along the way I hope to enable you to be independent in maintaining your optimal physical & mental state.

This exercise is part of the process...
For this exercise make a list of the foods you will be eating for the coming week.

You can then use this list, or pass it to whoever does your shopping, to buy the foods you require in advance.

Pre-planning & shopping for meals helps you stick to a defined menu.

It begins with knowing what you should & should not be eating, depending on your goal. I will have helped you refine this from Principles 15 & 16.

By completing this exercise you'll be shopping well, providing a greater potential for cooking well, eating well & ultimately feeling, looking & performing well.

All of these things take you one step closer to being in your optimal state.

Once you have thought through your entire week of eating you will realise how much food you consume in a week, or how little food you consume if you are not eating enough.

It may take only one run through this exercise to create a shift in your thinking around meal times.

Once you experience something, you learn from it, you cannot then unlearn it.

It's installed - imprinted in your brain forever.

The idea of this exercise is to transition your thoughts around meals from only thinking about your next meal to thinking more long-term. Each meal impacts you. Whether that impact is positive or negative is your choice.

You will know that from whatever line of business you are in, or wherever you have taken your career up to this point, that long-term planning is a way of increasing your likelihood of success.

The same principle applies to your eating, nutritional intake & management of your health.

You would be wise to limit your sugar intake. Remember from earlier that fresh fruit is good for you but in moderation.

Follow the guidelines I have provided you from Principles 14 & 15.

Plan ahead…
You will have most likely heard the saying - fail to prepare &
prepare to fail.
This is an accurate description of potential events. However you are
in control of the outcome of the forthcoming events – its all a mater
of choice.

Set up a table similar to the one below & sketch out an outline of
your meals for the week:

Monday	Tuesday	Wednesday	Thursday	Friday	Saturday	Sunday
Breakfast:	Breakfast:	Breakfast:	Breakfast:	Breakfast:	Breakfast:	Breakfast:
Snack:	Snack:	Snack:	Snack:	Snack:	Snack:	Snack:
Lunch:	Lunch:	Lunch:	Lunch:	Lunch:	Lunch:	Lunch:
Snack:	Snack:	Snack:	Snack:	Snack:	Snack:	Snack:
Dinner:	Dinner:	Dinner:	Dinner:	Dinner:	Dinner:	Dinner:
Beverages:	Beverages:	Beverages:	Beverages:	Beverages:	Beverages:	Beverages:

Here is an example of what Monday could look like:

Monday

Breakfast:	Snack:	Lunch:	Snack:	Dinner:	Beverages:
4 poached eggs, Grilled Steak, Mushrooms, Tomatoes, Onions, Peppers.	Celery, Cottage cheese or Quark	Grilled Chicken, Steamed Broccoli, Green beans & Carrots	Protein shake or one Apple Or juiced vegetables	Grilled Turkey breast, Boiled Cauliflower Cabbage & Peas.	Tea Coffee Milk /rice milk/ almond milk, semi skimmed or full fat?

Remember to proportion your meal sizes to the guidelines I
provided a little earlier. For instance you may eat two chicken
breasts if your daily requirements determine that.

Principle 20
I Plan For Optimal Eating In Advance

Remember to follow the meal coaching I provided you earlier. Apply Principles 15 & 16 daily. Before long you will begin to see & feel the positive effects of living by these principles.

These principles help you structure the amount you eat in a day, how much of each food you consume at each meal & ultimately the size of each meal & snack.

Only when you truly grasp how to manage this area of your life will you be in full control of your body shape & your performance – mentally as well as physically.

Sticking to a way of eating that brings about your optimal state requires some forethought & planning.

Like anything new, at first it may appear like a chore, but with a little practice you'll notice that the effort is well worth the reward & after a while you'll make smart choices without having to think about it.

This is a big step toward your long-term continued success. You would have heard the saying 'Fail to prepare & prepare to fail'. This is true. However, you now know exactly what needs to be in your plan.

Go ahead & plan your success.

Solution 4: Supplementation

Chapter 13:
Your Personal Supplements

50,000–63,000 individuals in the United States and 19,000–25,000 in the UK die prematurely from cancer annually due to insufficient vitamin D.

—John Cannell, MD

Supplementation is one of those controversial subjects that people struggle to process because there are so many conflicting views on the subject.

Your main nutrients & health should come from food this is the thought held by most people without argument.

However what also needs to be taken into consideration is any damage to your body from an 'un-healthy diet', either in the past or currently & nutrient deficiencies from your current lifestyle, exercise & nutrition patterns.

On top of that, can you honestly answer that you eat perfectly & that you eat whole foods that are super-rich in nutrients 100 percent of the time?

On top of that, the nutrient content of the food we eat is not as high as it used to be—so we are not getting as many nutrients by default[1]

---

1 http://hortsci.ashspublications.org/content/44/1/15.full

Supplementation is still one of the best ways to help your body restore itself & fix those little deficiencies that hold you back, make you ill & halt even greater success—both on a mental & physical level.

The name explains how they should be used—to *supplement* your already healthy, high-nutrient diet & lifestyle.

The Malice of Modern Diets

I am not a nutritionist, herbalist, or doctor.

These are my personal opinions, based on the specialised coaching, recommended training, diet & supplements I have provided to my clients through the years. I also regularly work with nutritionists & doctors to fine-tune people's requirements.

I have studied under highly qualified people within this field & have learned a lot from some very smart teachers. I apply what I learn, keeping what works & discarding what doesn't. What follows is my personal experiences & understanding of these matters.

Everyone is different. Just as you cannot expect a doctor to know what is happening inside your body after a fifteen-minute appointment, you cannot expect me to diagnose you from the ground up psychically!

Supplementation is about knowledge, testing, re-testing & regular adjustment.

Disorders, unpleasant side effects & even disease (like diabetes) may have taken root, caused by poor lifestyle & eating habits, among other things.

It is extremely common & therefore extremely likely that you have some kind of vitamin deficiency. Most people live with deficiencies for most of their lives, not fully aware of how removing that deficiency could dramatically improve their life.[1]

Vitamin & mineral deficiencies can be so subtle that the symptoms you experience may not be diagnosed as a problem. They can also be so severe that they are mistaken for another disease or illness.

As you will now be aware, when you lack one vitamin, it throws off your body's natural balance. Then it becomes impossible for you to be at your personal best.

Whatever the case, know your blood chemistry well & make sure you are not living with *any* deficiencies.

After all, if you are deficient in any way, how can you possibly be at your best?

Why Supplementation Is Needed

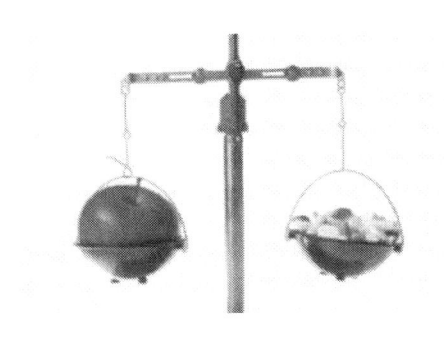

Food is fuel. Depending on your choice of food it can also be poison... or a medicine.

If you want to thrive—not just survive—then being at your peak requires feeding your body exactly what it needs & making sure you are consistent with that type of eating.

---

1 http://www.cdc.gov/media/releases/2012/p0402_vitamins_nutrients.html

Here is the unencumbered truth:

- Evidence from the National Diet & Nutrition Survey shows that the UK population does not achieve nutritional sufficiency through diet alone.

- Executive secretary of the UK Council for Responsible Nutrition said that recent NHS findings that diet alone is enough were flawed. She went on to say, "I am a little surprised that the NHA did not refer to [their own] data."

Your body needs supplementation because:

- *There are not enough nutrients in our food to cover our requirements.*
  Perhaps we did have enough decades ago, but mass-produced, intensive growing methods & farming practices leave fruits & vegetables with significantly fewer nutrients than people think.[1]

- *The age of our food must also be taken into consideration.*
  How old is that bunch of apples you bought yesterday? Eating food that is a week, two weeks, or even a month old is not eating fresh, high-nutrient food. If you're eating a South African apple & you live in London, it obviously wasn't picked yesterday. The older the food, the lower its nutritional value.[2]

- *Poor food preparation*
  Not only is the food lower quality, but we also use cooking processes like microwaves & high-oil heat

---

1 http://www.scientificamerican.com/article/soil-depletion-and-nutrition-loss/

2 http://www.foodrenegade.com/your-apples-year-old/

cooking that remove whatever nutrients are left, denature the food & end up eating fats that do use harm.

Did you know that over cooking your vegetables (& food in general) removes vital nutrients & digestive enzymes. Ultimately this means that your body has less access to the nutrients it needs to be at optimal & on top of that cannot absorb the nutrients does get access to.[1]

- ***Poor food digestion***
Your body needs high-quality nutrients to function optimally—but you can't absorb these nutrients because the modern diet causes damage to your digestive tract, which diminishes nutrient uptake.

On top of that as mentioned above, some cooking processes reduce the absorption rate of foods due to the loss of digestive enzymes. As with everything there is a balance. Some foods require cooking or you will poison yourself, chicken is a good example. However, over cooking certain foods will reduce your vitality. First step is to become aware of your options & the result of the cooking methods on the food you consume.

Off-the-Charts Toxicity Levels

If you can spare a moment to dismiss soil depletion, water pollution, poor animal rearing, battery-cage farms & consider poor cooking practices, there is still the horror of toxin exposure to deal with.

You need nutrients to deal with the toxins you are exposed to every day. The more toxins in the environment, the more nutrients you need for detox & healing.

---

1 http://www.ncbi.nlm.nih.gov/pubmed/15342442

In tests done in the United States on non-industry workers (teachers, journalists), they were found to have one hundred toxins in their bodies that were not present forty years ago.

Things to consider

- **Hormones**, pesticides & antibiotics in your meat & food negatively affect your body's ability to regulate itself. Nowadays the use of pesticides, growth hormone & antibiotics is common practice.

  Certain hormones can make young animals gain weight faster. They help reduce the waiting time & the amount of feed eaten by an animal before slaughter in meat industries. In dairy cows, hormones can be used to increase milk production. Therefore increasing profitability

  In turn we get a taste of these chemicals & hormones when we consume the food they have been administered on. There may not be enough toxins in one meal to kill you, however it would be logical to assume that regular consumption has to create a build up within your system. This is one more reason to eat organic.

- **Xenoestrogens** (foreign estrogens, that mimic estrogen), plastics like BPA (found in plastic water bottles), petroleum & dozens of other toxins that we come into contact with daily.[1]

- **Industrial solvents** & cleaners in grocery store shopping aisles & house cleaning products expose the average person to highly toxic chemicals that

---

1 http://www.dailymail.co.uk/health/article-2157423/Poisoned-plastic-Chemicals-water-bottles-food-packaging-linked-infertility-birth-defects-Scaremongering-truth.html

linger on furniture & in the air & also get into your body through your skin & the food you eat.

- **_Dry-cleaning procedures._** Chemicals used to clean your clothes have been found to be highly toxic.[1,2]

The full effects of the above mentioned chemicals & additional hormones on or in the human body is unknown. There are approximately 100 new chemicals added to our food supply each year. These chemicals are not known for their health giving properties! In fact, most of them are known for the opposite of improving health.

They disrupt the natural function of your body & the balance of your hormones creating adverse reactions to everyday life in the form of physical & emotional reactions to what appear to be everyday stimulus.

The vast list of potential poisons could arguably play a role in the onset of depression for some people. For instance: mercury fillings for teeth, food poisoning, solvents & the array of hormones, food additives, pesticides & fungicides must all have their impact on your health.

It is argued that the pesticides, fungicides & insect repellents yield higher crop returns, which in most cases may be true, but in that process do we lose quality at the expense of quantity?

Do the foods hold lower nutritional values? Do they poison you by containing a cocktail of hormones & insect repellent chemicals? The big question must be, is there a better way?

For no, let's just agree that we live in highly toxic environments.

---

1 http://www.webmd.com/cancer/news/20100209/dry-cleaning-chemical-likely-causes-cancer

2 http://www.naturalnews.com/023365_health_cleaning_dry.html

When you exercise, you need more nutrients to recover, heal & grow.

Your body desperately requires specific proportions of vitamins & minerals to give it a chance of maintaining your fast-paced lifestyle.

This is critical information if you want to live in an optimal state, if you want to achieve your personal best.

If you have been feeling under the weather, or your energy levels are not what they used to be, then vitamin & mineral inadequacies could be the root, or at least a large proportion of the problem.

If you want to get to the top & remain there, follow the principles outlined in this book.

"Healthy body - healthy mind" is an accurate statement. The opposite can also be applied, the more mental cleaning you do, keeping your mind clean, healthy & vital the better chance your body will have as you will make choices that are wiser & more positive.

Poison your mind through the methods mentioned above & your body will certainly suffer.

Are You Eating Enough to Be Nourished?

I am a big proponent of shopping for strictly organic food & preparing it in ways that conserve its nutritional value. But even if I do this every day, there's still a good chance I won't be taking in a perfect blend of nutrients specific to my unique requirements.

No diet is perfect. Just like a training program requires regular adjustment to maintain or develop greater fitness, your diet requires adjustment to provide your body with exactly what it needs.

The Principles of Optimalism are about a completely balanced body, mind & spirit.

The way to consciously achieve this is to follow the suggestions I have made throughout this book. Within that process you will determine & discovery many things about yourself.

No one can eat enough nutrients 100 percent of the time. You most likely have a hectic schedule & there will be times when you cannot help but skip a meal, or do not have a healthy choice available for a day or more.

If this happens, your body will not have the nutrients to keep it at peak physical condition. Your body will suffer & so will your performance & mind—especially if this happens every week, or several times a week. This is very common.

As a result, you wont be able to repair, detox & grow optimally. Your cravings for certain foods may increase, as your body desperately needs nourishment. This is when most people fail their new health & fitness plans & slip back into old eating habits.

At this point most people become despondent & return to previous habits. Prevent yourself from making this mistake by understanding that food is not the only way to get the nutrients that your body needs.

Supplements (well chosen) will help you.

Your Blood Never Lies

I prefer to take a clinical approach to vitamin & mineral deficiencies. Your blood can help you find out where you need to plug the nutrient gaps in your diet.

Your Blood Doesn't Lie.

Visit any GP & request a blood test for nutrient or vitamin deficiencies. This clinical process is quick & painless. It simply involves drawing & analysing your blood.

If your GP refuses, you may have to get this done privately. I have my own system that I walk clients through, explaining everything along the way.

If you live in London you can find my private blood screening through my website. I use a 12 Week Supplementation Program (12WSP) form of implementation.

Once you have the benchmark, you can take specific action. If deficiencies are present (this is very common) either your doctor or the lab you had the tests with will go through your best course of action. Otherwise source a professional who can handle this with you.

Once your blood chemistry is right, you'll notice a massive improvement in your health, level of performance, productivity, clarity of mind & sleep, to name only a few important improvements.

Also, your body-shaping results will accelerate.

You'll drop fat like never before, gain muscle easier than ever—basically, you'll eliminate the factors that have been blocking you for most of your life.

Most importantly, you will feel free; you will feel *more alive.*

Principle Exercise 21
Your Blood Never Lies

3Do you know the levels of vitamins & minerals within your
blood?
Do you know for sure that you are optimally nourished?

If you are deficient in any vitamin or mineral then there is no way
that
you can be in an optimal state.

It's like building a car with a part or a number of parts missing,
or using inferior parts that most definitely affect the overall
performance of the car.

When you are lacking in a vitamin or mineral, all of the functions
that it supports will be negatively affected.

You cannot expect optimal performance when you are draining
your system due to insufficient nutrient uptake.

Taking a supplement is like taking out health insurance for your
body. You are supporting the internal functions of your system in
order to bring about higher performance levels on the outside.

Don't allow any form of deficiency to hold you back if there is
something you can do about it.

Get your blood tested & know your nutritional status. Then take
the necessary steps to optimalise your blood.

I highly advise that you work with a professional to complete this process. This is not the type of thing where you take a lone ranger approach. You need an expert to guide you.

If you live in London:
Go to my website: www.ShapeTrainer.co.uk

Now press 12WSP (12Week-Supplementation-Program)
Here you'll read the process of my twelve-week program.

You can book yourself in online, right there, right away.

Principle 21
I Maintain Optimal Nutrients Within My Blood

It is critically important that you have a full nutritional evaluation (blood tests to determine the nutritional status of your blood) at least once every year.

This way you can stay on top of your health in an accurate & effective way.

Once you know your blood, it will shed some light on

where you have been stopped in the past.

You will likely break through plateaus, smash personal bests, achieve

your lowest & healthiest body fat percentage ever.

The aim of this entire book is to help you create the very best version of yourself.

Getting to know your blood is an essential part of that process.

Perfect your blood chemistry & watch your success rates soar —physically, mentally & emotionally.

If you ever feel under par or not quite your best or you feel that something is holding you back from performing at 100 percent – this could hold the answer.

Maintaining optimum nutrients within your blood & keeping yourself in peak condition is a master key to unlocking your full potential.

Branded

When it comes to supplements it is important you make the right choice of brand. Not all supplements are made equal. Not all supplements contain the best ingredients. Not all supplements are proportioned optimally.

I use a brand that I trust & have been using for many rears now. It is critically important that you ingest the best quality of supplement as possible. They may cost you a little more but the extra investment will be well worth it.

In the long run you will get better results, be healthier & actually save money. Talk to professionals that you know & trust to get recommendations.

If you follow my recommendation & have your blood tested then your next steps are:

- Take the supplements & vitamins daily that you need to fix your deficiencies.

- Take note of how you feel & adjust accordingly over the coming weeks.

- In three to six months, return for another blood test to see how your levels have improved. After your retest, adjust your supplementation accordingly.

Your body wants to be healthy, so once you begin providing it exactly what it needs you will see an immediate improvement.

I have witnessed many of my clients' old aches, issues & pains vanish after they have corrected their vitamin deficiencies. I strongly advise you to consider this process.

Special Note

Taking blood & supplementing your diet should be conducted under the supervision of an expert. Do not guess or take supplements blindly.

Follow the professional guidelines from clinical studies for supplementation. Follow the advice of a skilled professional.

Source a respected, trustworthy professional & pay the expert to guide you through the process. It will be one of the best investments you have ever—& will ever—make.

Formulating a Supplement Plan

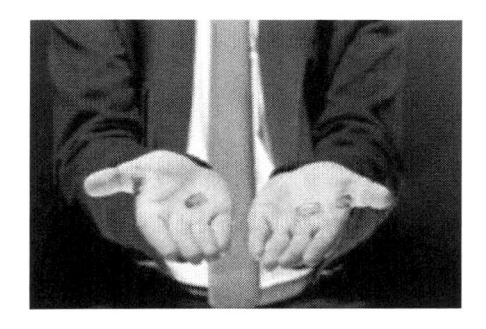

Your supplement plan will be formulated once you receive your blood tests & have a platform to work from.

Then you'll treat, or supplement, the levels in your body. Remember, the recommended daily allowance represent what we need to *survive*.

If you're starting at a deficit, you need a little extra to get you back to where you're supposed to be. It will need to be this way for a period of time in order to bring you levels back to optimum.

This is especially true when you treat a disease or disorder. Also bear in mind that the expert you work with should expose what caused the deficiency in the first place in order to ensure it doesn't keep you deficient.

In this particular situation, survival levels of supplementation may not help you. Higher doses will be therapeutic at this point. Again, each case is unique & that is why I strongly suggest having your blood chemistry determined through testing with a professional.

This way you know exactly what you are doing, why you are doing it & how long you should do it for.

When you receive your test results, sit down & chat with your professional coach about the supplements & vitamins you can take to improve your health.

Important Steps:

- Create your supplement plan based on your blood-test results.

- The first step of the plan will be to find the right brand & take the supplements for a week or so to notice any immediate effects.

Record your findings in a fitness journal to help you keep track of your physical & medical progress. Or simply use the notes on your phone.

A simple system is emoticons. A sad, neutral, or smiley face indicates your mental, physical & emotional state at three points during the day.

I have seen within two weeks of applying a supplementation protocol, the emoticon chart can go from mostly sad to mostly happy symbols.

Simply being happy is the foundation for feeling satisfied about your life. Optimising your vitamin & mineral levels brings about more frequent feelings of contentment & reduces feelings of stress & frustration[1, 2]

For example, those who are severely deficient in magnesium will be hyper-reactive to stress, which compounds into more stressful situations[3]

Handle the magnesium deficiency & there will be less reaction when stressful situations arise in your life & therefore less overall stress—not to mention less fat around your middle & a better night's sleep.

1 http://www.mentalhealth.org.uk/help-information/mental-health-a-z/D/diet/

2 http://greatist.com/happiness/nutrients-boost-mood

3 http://www.ncbi.nlm.nih.gov/pubmed/25373528

Principle Exercise 22
Emoticon Chart

See below for an example of a weekly emoticon chart.

Use this to track your mood & mental state.

Within each circle draw a face that matches your mood; smiley face, neutral face or sad face. Do this in the morning, at lunchtime & in the evening.

At the end of the day note your average mood for the day. For instance, two smiley faces would suggest a predominantly positive day so draw a happy face as the average for that day.

If you have an unhappy face for the morning, neutral face for lunch & a smiley face for evening then apply a neutral face for the average of that day.

Date:	Morn	Afternoon	Evening	Day Average
MONDAY	○	○	○	○
TUESDAY	○	○	○	○
WEDNESDAY	○	○	○	○
THURSDAY	○	○	○	○
FRIDAY	○	○	○	○
SATURDAY	○	○	○	○
SUNDAY	○	○	○	○

Principle 22
I Understand And Effectively Manage My Mood

Having a basic or comprehensive understanding about your mood patterns, what affects them, what situations, people or food create specific moods is essential if you want to master optimal living.

Only when you first acknowledge the situation/condition can you then do something about it.

For instance, a similar emoticon chart was used by athletes to determine if they were over training. In the morning the athlete would make a note of their overall state by drawing a face. This proved to be an accurate assessment of the physical condition of the athlete, even when compared to state of the art testing.

You are looking for a clear sign of improvement over passing weeks.

As you apply more & more of the principles within this book, you'll notice a subtle shift for the positive.

How you are affected by different stimulus will become clear, & this will show up through the emoticon chart. You could have reactions from a meal, from supplements, from a late night etc.

Make notes on the chart if you get headaches or feel tired or exceptionally happy or unhappy. Note any positive or negative experiences.

Do this every week so that in two months' time, you have eight charts to compare.
Once you see patterns then you can begin to make changes to your supplement plan, eating habits, sleep times or even the amount of time you spend with certain people.

***If you follow the principles within this book,
you will see improvements.***

*It is an important element for continued success that you clearly see
your progress.
An improvement in mood could mean an improvement in
performance, mentally & physically.*

*An improvement in mood could indicate that your level of health is
improving. It could help to improve relationships, both personal &
business.*

*The other side of this is that if you are consistently getting unhappy
faces through your days then it is clear that something needs to be
addressed.*

*The principles up to this point will help you structure which areas
of your life that could need further detailed attention. Be honest
with yourself as to how closely you are following each principle of
Optimalism.*

*It could be your thoughts, your sleeping patterns, eating habits,
your water intake or fluid intake, your exercise plan or lack of, or it
could be the supplements or lack of supplements that is the problem.*

*Whatever your personal case, the structure I have set up will help
guide you toward a more optimal state of being.*

*Once you begin to apply more of the principles along side each other
you will generate exponential growth. This means that if you look
at each principle in isolation you may initially think that it will not
have much impact.*

*However when you apply two or three or four of the principles
throughout consecutive days you will notice a more dramatic shift.
The rate of improvement can be sped up.*

Over time, after repeatedly living through these principles you will build a momentum. This momentum will also increase in speed & strength the longer you continue the pattern that initiated it.

Like a train with forward momentum it becomes very hard to stop, even if obstacles appear along the way your momentum will help you smash through those barriers.

Even if you stop applying a principle or two, everything that you had built up will not be lost.

This is where a short break in taking supplements, or eating a meal that you know is unhealthy will not cause you much or any concern. You can get away with more. As long as you return to 'what works' shortly after you will keep your momentum in the positive direction.

So begin to understand what works & what doesn't. Begin to have a deeper understanding of yourself & repeatedly do that which makes you healthier & fitter.

This is your concern, your main focus... after which everything else will fall into place.

Chapter 14:
Missing Nutrient X

"Health is not valued till sickness comes"

Thomas Fuller
(English author & historian)

When you have a demanding career, you learn to live with things. I have seen many people live with aches, pains, tiredness, injury after injury & illness after illness. When you are overworked & undernourished you are running the risk of breakdown.

If you are not firing on all cylinders mentally & physically I have to ask you why?

What if I told you that finding "missing nutrient X" could stop many of those everyday symptoms. Many of my clients have done this & experienced incredible results.

Why Invest in Supplements?

Supplementation is an investment—in your body, in your health & in your future finances. Like with any medical field, you have to do your research first.

It's frustrating when people declare that vitamins don't work or supplementation is a rip-off when I have seen so much improvement in health—physically & mentally—with so many people over many years.

Of course supplements will not work for you if you rush out, uneducated & buy the cheapest, "nicest-looking" supplement you can find. Who knows if they are made from the best quality ingredients? You also have to know they are the right supplements for your specific needs.

Invest in quality. You should never cut corners with supplements. Researched supplementation is an investment in your physical, mental, financial, emotional & spiritual future. It can determine your level of success.

Without Your Health, You Have Nothing.

There is nothing more important than your health—& your health will never be at its peak as long as there is a lack of nutrients in your body.

Choose the Right Supplements to Enhance Wellness

The supplements you eventually choose will be based on your unique needs & physical condition.

They will enhance your overall wellness & make it easier for you to achieve the level of physical & mental performance you want.

They have the power to

- **Fix old deficiencies**: You may have a deficiency & not even know about it. A lack of vitamin D, for example causes bone softening, easy breaks, fatigue & "foggy" brain syndrome. These will all lift with appropriate vitamin D supplementation.

- **Increase your body's healing power**: When you have the right nutrients for training, it dramatically helps the fat loss & muscle building processes & massively decreases your chances of getting injured. When you improve your vitamin & mineral levels, you heal quicker—from muscle soreness to a cut on your finger.

The whole point of the Optimalism is to get you to peak physical condition without putting you on a ridiculous regimen of pills & potions.

What I achieve with my clients is a detailed, individualised program of high-quality food & high-quality specific supplements. You want to be you—just even better.

That means you must plan the supplements you choose & they need to be proven effective.

Dosage & Time Considerations

Once you have identified the supplements you want to take, there's only one thing left to do—determine the dosage & treatment regimen.

Quick Tips

- **Each person requires a unique amount of each vitamin & mineral.** Your blood is the most accurate way to determine how much & for how long you require each nutrient to remain in an optimal state.

- **Get more than one opinion.** Your doctor may not advocate supplementation, but your local pharmacist might. Talk to as many qualified people as possible to get a solid overview of supplementation & the specific approach that is right for you.

- **Read labels.** If the recommended dose is way off what you have been told, address it. Be aware that the recommended dose on the bottle may not be adequate to correct a deficiency. Again, work with a professional to determine what is safe for you.

- **Use studies.** Clinical studies can highlight effective or dangerous dosages of a substance. A collection of studies reaching the same conclusions would be a good guideline. Check out www.PubMed.com for one source of professional studies. The dosage results from these studies are invaluable information.

- **Reassess your status every twelve to sixteen weeks.** "Forever" is not a treatment regimen; it's an open-ended sales pitch. Regular blood tests—or at the very least, once a year—will help you.

Keep in mind that new supplements come out every day that may be an improvement on your current choice.

Do not get stuck on one supplement alone. If you find a brand that really works for you, stay up-to-date on the company's new product releases & the latest studies from respected sources.

The easiest way for a busy person to remain up-to-date with all this info is to closely follow a reliable expert. I send weekly emails & blogs to my mailing list, keeping them informed about the latest relevant information.

One of the easiest ways to get your hands on condensed info is to locate a great health practitioner. A trusted professional can filter massive amounts of data & deliver the most appropriate & effective information directly to you.

All of this info is set to inform you & speed up your health & fitness results/progress. I filter information for my clients so they don't have to. I remain up-to-date so they don't have to. The info I provide will save them time & energy.

Make sure your expert is knowledgeable. There are a lot of Internet experts who can "talk the talk" but do not "walk the walk" or have the results to back up what they say!

Documenting a Reaction

You may not think so, but supplements can have serious effects on your body. They are like medicine—they become *part* of your body & can systematically treat physical ailments & boost your immune system.[1]

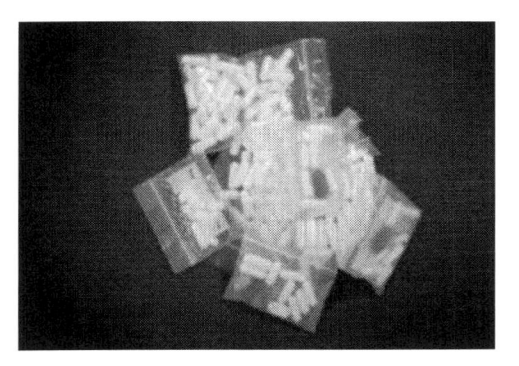

In many ways, this makes them more important than traditional medication as type of pre-medicine that wards off disease before it can take hold.

Remember–you are what you eat. The same can be said about your supplements. You health & performance will be influenced by the nutrients you ingest.

Using supplements intelligently is one of the best ways to avoid disease & illness. It's also an extremely effective way to speed up your results in the gym or with your chosen sport.

---

1 http://www.ncbi.nlm.nih.gov/pubmed/24281460

That's why I recommend that my clients record their mood & experiences in a journal or by using the emoticon chart from Principle 21.

Or you can do this simply with a note on your phone. Making a quick note of your mood throughout each day. After a few days you'll notice a pattern. When you have this data you can then take steps to do something about it.

Knowing & understanding your body on a micro-level will help you connect with it, nurture it & treat it as soon as something appears to be going wrong.

Not All Supplements Are Made Equal

All supplements will cause some kind of physical reaction in your body. The quality of the ingredients varies greatly from brand to brand & even batch to batch.

Don't cut corners with supplements. Search for the best, highly respected, trusted, highest quality source & use that supplement. It's well worth the small additional cost in the long run.

In fact, you'll save money by investing in quality from the outset.

The supplements will take effect quicker; you'll restore your nutrient levels quicker & therefore cut back on the dosing quicker.

You'll eliminate adverse reactions that can be brought on by cheaper ingredients & you'll perform better & enjoy your life more.

Exercise 23
Quality Border Control

From this moment on attempt to improve the quality of what you consume.

I'm talking supplements, food, beverages, visual images & even words & music.

Everything you consume or ingest or absorb impacts you.

All I am suggesting here is to slightly lift (in a positive sense) everything that enters your body, either through your mouth, through absorption on your skin, through your vision (what you watch or allow yourself to gaze at) or your ears - the type of music you listen to may be aggressive or negative? If so, raise the positivity for a few days & see if you notice a difference in your mood & performance.

One way to become more aware of your reactions & the outcome of these reactions over your life is to complete this simple exercise:

Take two minutes every evening to record how your supplements & diet make you feel physically, mentally & emotionally.

You can also do this twenty minutes after you eat & take your supplements, record how you feel mentally, physically & emotionally.

- ***Make notes of things like:***

My mind feels sharp.
or
My mind feels fuzzy & slow.

My energy levels are through the roof
or
I have little energy & want to go to sleep!

I feel happy & calm
or
I feel angry, agitated & reactive.

…You get the point.

Once you have completed this exercise for several days in a row you'll have some data about yourself & your current patterns.

You can apply this technique to any area of your life. How does the music you listen to make you feel twenty or so minutes after your listening time?

Apply this process to any area of your life that you want to assess. This will inform you if you are on track rather than blocking your way to an optimal state of being.

Once you can acknowledge the positivity or negativity of something you can then choose to do more of it or less of it – the choice is yours.

Principle 23
I Only Ingest Substances That Increase My Vitality

This principle applies to every area of your life & not just supplements.

To align yourself with the best produce at every meal, alongside the best supplements will boost your health toward the best version of itself – which supports the best version of yourself.

The same goes for whatever you choose to assess in your life, take the music example from above, once you have highlighted the music that brings about a higher state of being for you it becomes another tool to project you in the direction of success.

You'll already be aware that when you demand the best you more often get the best – out of people, from hotels, from restaurants etc.

So always source the best supplements & only use the trusted brand or brands that you know. Listen to the right music for you, use the best lotion/shampoo/aftershave etc.

One of your goals is to become aware of your mental, physical & emotional reactions to everything you consume.

You may eat food & supplements, but they affect your mind & mood as well as your stomach.

From Principle 21 you will already be more aware of what lifts you & what deflates you.
Cut back on what deflates you. Effectively manage what lifts you.

What you'll become more sensitive to is the subtle impact of each meal & each supplement, each training session, each sleep & each thought etc.

What you put in will determine what you get out.

Only putting in the best will increase your chances of only producing high quality performance - mentally & physically.

You are now beginning to refine optimal living & are one step closer to Living Through Optimalism.

Chapter 15:
Supplement Overview

Take care of your body with steadfast fidelity. The soul must see through these eyes alone, and if they are dim, the whole world is clouded.

—*Goethe*

All supplements are different & cause various responses in different people.

To accurately know how one will react in your body:

i. Trust your healthcare professional
ii. Follow your blood test results
iii. Stick to a respected & trusted supplement company

Below is a quick overview of *my personal* baseline supplement regime. This is not set to diagnose you & I am certainly not telling you to start taking these supplements right now.

You must follow individualised professional guidance designed for you.

It is your choice what information you decide to apply to your life.

Having said that, the following is the baseline supplements that I advise my clients to invest in as soon as possible.

Taking a Multivitamin

There has been a lot of chatter bad-mouthing multivitamin supplements & this talk has some merit.

There are lots of companies that follow their own protocols, create inferior products, add extra or non-health promoting ingredients in order to increase profit margins. There are numerous studies that have found a contradiction from what is on the bottle to what is actually within the product.

This problem can cause the supplement to appear inferior or to have no positive effect. Which can then be used as a basis for the argument that supplements do no promote health.

This however, is an issue of company morality & procedure rather than actual cause & effect of taking specific doses of certain supplements to help alleviate or cure ailments.

In short, the supplement may not be the issue. It could be the dosage, or the quality of the ingredient(s), age of the supplement or biological requirements of the individual.

Here is what you need to know about multivitamin supplements:

- *Good multivitamins help your body maintain balance* so that it can function at its best. They complement a busy life, help you stay on top of things at work & promote overall health, physically & mentally. They do this by keeping your micronutrients closer to optimal levels.

- *Studies prove that people who take a daily multivitamin live, on average, five years longer than those who do not.*[1]

---

1 http://www.ncbi.nlm.nih.gov/pubmed/19279081

- ***How do you choose?*** Look for certifications & FDA approval & do not buy the cheapest or the most expensive. Rather, source them based on advice, referrals & research through word-of-mouth, face-to-face & online. Gain the advice of a respected professional rather than a random online expert who could be drumming up sales based on commission.

- ***How much do you take?*** Ask your doctor, read the label & most importantly follow your lab results.

- ***How long do you take it for?*** Ask your doctor, check your performance levels & again follow lab results to remain at optimal levels. On average, a lot of people take one to three multivitamins a day for life.

- ***Benefits include increased productivity.*** They will help you *look* your best, enjoy higher energy levels, greater clarity & sharpness of mind & your sex drive could also improve over time.

- ***Multis give you a little top up.*** They are insurance for your health & vitality. They can help support you in times of high stress & erratic eating or boost you in times of perfect lifestyle & sports performance.

- ***I instantly recommend a multi to my clients.*** I only recommend the brand I supply, as I am 100 percent confident in its quality.

- ***I have my clients start on these as soon as possible.*** One a day can be enough, but keeping your vitamin levels topped up is one of the easiest & wisest things you can do. It is in effect taking out an insurance policy on your health.

Taking Amino Acids

Amino acids are used to build muscle, detoxify & repair the cells of your body.

This is what you need to know about amino acid supplementation:

- *Good amino acid supplements should come in a bioavailable form,* this means that most if not the entire dose you take actually enters your circulatory system. For instance, intravenous injections are 100% bioavailable. Generally, amino acids come in vegetable capsules or gel/liquid caps or powder, which you dissolve in liquid & drink.

- *How do you choose?* Look for amino acids containing the essential three: valine, leucine & isoleucine. Ask at your local gym—there will be lots of members who have taken different brands. I recommend the brand that is available through my website.

- *How much do you take?* Ask your doctor, read the label & follow your lab reports. You need your lab or health practitioner to test you for their version of an amino-acid-profile blood test. There is a science behind how much you should take for your body weight. Again, a good health professional can provide you with this calculation.

- *How long do you take it for?* It depends on your goals. If you want to build a lot of muscle from the beginning, take them until you reach your target. Then stop, or switch to a maintenance dose. Your blood can determine the answer to this question.

Generally speaking, amino acids are great to take every time you train.

- ***Benefits include preventing the breakdown of muscle tissue during intense exercise.*** They also naturally increase production of human growth hormone & contribute to stronger, leaner muscle tone. They will speed up your results from training & help you recover quicker.

- ***Natural food sources:*** Eggs, meat, fish, cottage cheese are rich in protein. You can also come by protein & amino acids in the form of healthy, natural shakes or drinks. Be sure the source is respected, or you could be ingested something that aggravates you & stunts your progress.

- *S*ome other benefits of taking amino acid supplementation:

  - *Require no digestion. Therefore can be absorbed directly into your blood stream as a pure source of protein.*
  - Increase speed of recovery from exercise
  - Increase fat burning potential, particularly visceral fat (organ)
  - Improve the use of glucose throughout the body
  - Increase Insulin sensitivity
  - A direct source of energy while you train or endure a busy day

- *R*emember: Principle 23 - Only Ingest The Best

Taking Fish Oil

It is common knowledge that fish oil can help with heart issues, protection against heart disease & even lower the risk of Alzheimer's. Alongside being a natural anti-inflammatory.

Fish oil is a good source of omega 3. Within the current average diet we consume too much omega 6. Omega6 is obtained from oil such as soybean, corn, borage & vegetable oils. They are commonly found in processed foods.

Most omega6 fatty acids *promote inflammation (while omega3 reduces inflammation)* & the typical American diet tends to contain on average 15-25 times more omega6 to omega3.[1]

This overconsumption of one type of omega wreaks havoc throughout your body & causes imbalance, especially if not addressed for prolonged periods of time.

On top of which, it is common these days for someone to be deficient in omega 3.

The American Heart Association recommends two servings a week of fatty fish rich in omega-3 as this will help reduce the rate of cardiac events in people with cardiovascular disease[2]Could this same recommendation be used to ward of heart disease?

You may also be aware of the different types of fish oil - omega 3, 6 & 9 are the most commonly heard of, but not forgetting omega 7. Each plays a vital role in the ability of your body & brain to deliver peak performance.

---

1 http://umm.edu/health/medical/altmed/supplement/omega3-fatty-acids

2 http://www.heart.org/HEARTORG/GettingHealthy/NutritionCenter/HealthyDietGoals/
   Fish-and-Omega-3-Fatty-Acids_UCM_303248_Article.jsp

According to the Nutrition Business Journal, fish oil products generated about \$1.2 billion in sales in the United States in 2013 & global sales are set to grow to \$3.3 billion by the year 2020 due to increased human consumption as the awareness of health benefits rise.[3]

That's a lot of fish oil being consumed, so there must be some benefits – right?

As always, if you want to experience optimal function of your body & brain, a balance is required. These days the average person does not consume enough fish oil to maintain an optimal state of being.

There have been links made with the ingestion of omega fatty acids & brain health. As your brain is the fattest organ in your body & can be made up of as much as 60% fat, it could be argued that pure sources of healthy fatty acids will help to maintain or improve healthy brain function.

A study within the Archives of General Psychiatry showed that America has the highest rate of bipolar disorder (4.4%). Whereas Japan for example showed low statistics of 0.7%[1]

Japan is one of the highest consumers of fish oil, as fish is a large portion of their natural diet. Even though they have similar work-life-balance to the US, could the increased consumption of fish oil be protecting their brains?

There are many studies that support the idea that fish oil improves health & helps prevent disease as presented below.

---

3 http://newhope360.com/breaking-news/global-fish-oil-market-reach-33-billion-2020-researchers-say

1 http://edition.cnn.com/2011/HEALTH/03/07/US.highest.bipolar.rates/

At time of writing these are the things we know:

- *Good fish oil supplements contain EPA & DHA in varying amounts,* depending on the blend & source. EPA stands for Eicosapentaenoic acid & is an omega3. DHA stands for Decosahexaenoic acid & is also an omega3. Both provide their own health benefits. You would be wise to rotate your blend of omega's to ensure you are covering all bases. For instance, one batch of supplement may hold a value of 6:1 (EPA:DHA), while another blend could be 1:10 (EPA:DHA). When supplementing it is also important to take into consideration the other omega's 6, 7 & 9. A health professional will structure a plan for you, this plan should be based on your blood work.

- *They should come in liquid or gel form.* These have been found to help improve body composition plus improve cardiovascular & metabolic health. When taken alongside a balanced diet & exercise program, the positive effects are increased.[2]

- *How do you choose?* Be brand aware; check that the supplement company uses ethical, local farming practices for extraction & passes all FDA regulations. Speak with as many people as possible & stay up to date with the latest info available. As mentioned earlier your health care professional should be able to point you in the right direction.

- *How much do you take?* Ask your doctor & read the label. Again your blood tests will provide a clearer indication of your specific requirements. As a rule of thumb, I recommend six grams a day to my clients.

This should be spread through the day: two grams at breakfast, two grams at lunch & two grams at dinner. If you follow my suggestion & have a full blood analysis to accurately tailor your plan you will notice an improvement in your results & overall level of health.

- ***You can take far beyond two to three grams per day, but the perfect amount for optimal health & physical performance depends on individual requirements.***

- ***How long do you take it for?*** You can take fish oil supplementation for life. Its benefits are well worth the investment. As mentioned earlier fish oil helps support a healthy heart & brain. If either of these two organs become dysfunctional so will your entire life – is it worth taking a little fish oil on a daily basis as an investment?

- ***Positive reasons to take fish oil:*** You can take fish oil to help reduce inflammation, balance your blood sugar, build muscle & ward off an endless list of diseases. Most experts recommend at least two to three grams of fish oil a day; some will go as high as thirty grams. Although large doses can cause excessive bleeding in some people, so it is best to work with a professional & base your intake on blood tests. The American Heart Association recommends a minimum of one gram per day.[1]

- ***Benefits are endless.*** Just Google "The health benefits of fish oil," & you will see what I mean. Benefits include a decrease in stress & anxiety, reduced inflammation, reduced signs of aging, protection

---

1 http://www.ncbi.nlm.nih.gov/pubmed/24954371

from pollutants, a boost in brain power & memory, lean muscle preservation, improved bone health & reduced chance of heart disease. Fish oil helps in the treatment of skin disorders & assists in muscle protein synthesis (growth of muscle), fat burning & insulin sensitivity…the list goes on.

- **Fish oil protects your brain:**
  Fish oil has also been found to slow the progress of Alzheimer's disease as mentioned earlier, so it is a natural brain protectant.[1]

- *Natural food sources:* Fish.

As long as you source the best quality fish & eat at least two meals containing that fish per week you should maintain healthy levels of omega3.

You'd be wise to supplement with fish oil as determined by your blood tests. Remember to rotate your blend (varying amounts of EPA to DHA as mentioned above), then you should be fine with taking fish oil supplements indefinitely.

I achieve this rotation of blends by selecting a different tub of fish oil once I complete my current one. All the options I use through my website are high quality & can be used for prolonged periods of time, if not indefinitely. Again, quality matters.

This is an important supplement that I instantly recommend to all my clients. It rapidly speeds results in every area & as soon as you start to supplement with fish you will notice mental & physical improvements—your performance will improve.

---

1 http://www.heart.org/HEARTORG/Encyclopedia/Heart-Encyclopedia_UCM_445084_Encyclopedia.jsp?levelSelected=6&title=fish%20oil

Taking Vitamin D3

It is estimated that 1 billion people worldwide are deficient in vitamin D.[1]

Numerous studies highlight that Vitamin D improves muscle efficiency & skeletal muscle functioning.[2,3]

Studies conducted by the Society for Endocrinology have also proved this to be true in 2013, presented at a conference in Harrogate, UK.

You may well know vitamin D as the bone vitamin. As it is commonly prescribed with calcium for those suffering with osteoporosis or similar bone density complications.

Vitamin D is one or more members of a group of steroid molecules. It is in fact a hormone precursor & therefore should give you an indication of how important its role is for optimal health.

You synthesise Vitamin D when your skin is exposed to direct sunlight. This is why it is not a true vitamin, as individuals with adequate exposure to sunlight do not require dietary supplementation.

You can of course use supplementation to maintain adequate levels for optimal health if you know you do not get enough sun & your blood results match that story.

As a lot of people now live an indoor lifestyle & wear more sunscreen than ever before because of the fear of skin cancer, we are left with a society deficient in this life-sustaining, bone building & immune boosting hormone.

---

1 http://www.ncbi.nlm.nih.gov/pubmed/20795941

2 http://www.ncbi.nlm.nih.gov/pubmed/24488588

3 http://www.ncbi.nlm.nih.gov/pubmed/24179588

Mood-D

D3 is linked to mood. Ever noticed how you feel much happier when you go on a summer holiday?

It could be due to the fact you are not at work or you're having a break from your usual routine, or that you're lying on a beautiful beach. In fact, a lot of that mood shift has to do with your body replenishing vitamin D3 stores from the sun[1]

For instance you will likely have heard about SAD (Seasonal Affective Disorder). A condition associated with the winter when there is less sunlight through the day. This coincides with a drop in D3 levels within the blood.

Every cell in your body has space for D3.

It should be present. If you have any sort of vitamin D3 deficiency, that means that every cell in your body is suffering from a deficiency which, depending on the extent of the deficiency, potentially exposes you to a number of conditions or disorders, SAD being one of them[2]

What this means is that you cannot possibly be at your best. You are capable of much more. Getting your blood work done & ensuring that your D3 levels are in an optimal state is essential if you want the best from your body & mind.

It also suggests that the closer to optimal your D3 stores the happier you will feel. Therefore, maintaining your D3 levels is a simple, worthwhile process in order to increase your experience of happiness.

---

1 http://www.ncbi.nlm.nih.gov/pubmed/23475735

2 http://www.ncbi.nlm.nih.gov/pubmed/9539254

Bone...

D3 also works synergistically (in combination) with magnesium & calcium. Two minerals associated with bone density.

When you get enough D3 from the sun, diet & supplementation you ward off bone density issues.[1]

In one study from the New England Journal of medicine it was clearly demonstrated that after 3 years of supplementing D3 & calcium both bone loss & fractures were decreased. Presenting the idea that D3 supports a healthy skeleton.[2]

One of the main functions of D3 is to maintain adequate crossing of substances across your cell membranes, thus enhancing the absorption & effectiveness of magnesium & calcium to your bones - among other vital nutrients.

It is important to note that without adequate stores of D3 you will not be able to absorb Calcium. So taking on board copious amounts of calcium to help support bone density is futile when your D3 stores are not optimal.

You're effectively taking Calcium into your blood but cannot get it into your cells where it is needed! Leaving your liver to process more substances out of your blood stream.

Health...

Aside from every cell (including your brain tissue) requiring D3, it is the only vitamin in the body that is actually a hormone.

1 http://www.ncbi.nlm.nih.gov/pubmed/23475735

2 http://www.ncbi.nlm.nih.gov/pubmed/9539254

Most people are aware these days of how much hormones play a role in overall health, mental & physical. When your hormones are out of whack so is the functioning of your body… & your life.

When a person drops out of equilibrium (balance) it is just a matter of time before they fall ill. In a lot of cases these days their immune system is so fatigued that it is no longer able to protect them. In fact it may be attacking them – as with autoimmune diseases.

The National Institute of Health (NIH) estimates that up to 23.5 million Americans have an autoimmune disease & this number is rising. In comparison, cancer affects up to nine million & heart disease up to twenty two million.[1]

Another extremely useful benefit of optimal D3 levels is an immune boosting potentiality.[2]

Several studies show that the closer to optimal your vitamin D levels within your blood, the better your body performs on every level.

One Harvard article highlights the prevalence of vitamin D deficiency, the latest research pointing to the importance of vitamin D supplementation, how vitamin D supports healthy bone, muscle, heart, immune function & can ward off disease including cancer, multiple sclerosis, diabetes, flu & colds… even reducing the risk of premature death.[3]

I'm sure you can now begin to see how important optimal levels of Vitamin D are.

From results I have experienced with my clients blood analysis, of applying supplementation to a healthy diet & exercise regime, I have seen

1 http://www.ncbi.nlm.nih.gov/pmc/articles/PMC3051848/

2 http://www.aarda.org/autoimmune-information/autoimmune-statistics/

3 http://www.hsph.harvard.edu/nutritionsource/vitamin-d/

many mental & physical improvements from supplementation (in this example D3).

Again, apply principle 21, test your blood & keep your levels within optimal range if you want to give yourself the best chance to reach & remain at your optimal state of being.

Reduced Risk To Cancer...

Breast, Prostate & Colorectal. Those with low levels of Vitamin D have an 83-150% increased risk of developing cancer.[1,2,3]

Within cancer cells it has been found that the vitamin D receptor is reduced. Having optimal receptor sites & then optimal stores has proven to regulate the cells more effectively, reduce inflammation & increase tumor cell death. [4,5]

Solid Tips

- *If you are from a country that sees more rain* than sunshine, then you most likely have a D3 deficiency.

- *Good vitamin D3 supplements ramp up the mitochondria power stations* of your body (energy production & optimal cell function), reduce muscle fatigue & lead to leaner, stronger muscles.

1 Bilinski K, Boyages J. Association between 25-hydroxyvitamin D concentration and breast cancer risk in an Australian population: an observational case-control study. Breast Cancer Res Treat. 2013 Jan;137(2):599-607

2 http://www.ncbi.nlm.nih.gov/pubmed/22508710

3 http://www.ncbi.nlm.nih.gov/pubmed/21724580

4 http://www.ncbi.nlm.nih.gov/pubmed/22939886

5 http://www.ncbi.nlm.nih.gov/pubmed/22801352

- D3 is one vitamin (hormone) that you cannot afford to be deficient in - that is, if you want to achieve your optimal state, if you want to get the best out of your body & mind.

- *Why is D3 so important? It is now known that nearly every cell within your body has a D3 receptor site.*

  This means that every cell in your body requires D3 to achieve an optimal state. If you have any level of D3 deficiency then it is impossible for you to be functioning at optimum. This means you cannot be delivering your full potential – you have even more to give.

  It is well known in the bodybuilding community that ramping up D3 will help muscle growth.

  Alongside looking better on stage, suntans are an essential part of a bodybuilders arsenal for the reasons explained above. We already know that D3 plays a role in optimal muscle contraction & bone health.

  Want more muscle? D3 will help you develop it. Obviously supplement in balance with your blood tests as over dosing on D3 holds some severe consequences (however unlikely for most people these days)

- *How do you choose?* Look for a bioavailable form in the recommended dose. Ask your doctor & follow your health care professional's advice.

- *How much do you take?* Ask your doctor, read the label, follow your blood reports. It has been reported that supplementing with two large doses per week is more effective at raising D3 levels from a deficient status.

But only attempt this with the supervision of a health care professional in line with your blood tests.

- *Overconsumption of a D3 supplement is highly dangerous. Follow a structured plan from a highly respected lab or health care professional.*

- *How long do you take it for?* If you have vitamin D deficiency & are prone to not getting enough sunlight, then take it for as long as you need it (your blood work determines this).

Another option is to get more sunlight on your skin. Allow as much of your skin to be exposed to the sunlight as possible, but be aware of time exposure & how strong the sunlight is to avoid burning. Use common sense, with the aim of getting sunlight on your skin.

- *Benefits include improved muscle performance,* less fatigue, more energy, increased bone density, an increase in an optimistic mood, better sleep, greater ability to relax & a host of other long-lasting contributing factors for better overall health.

- *Natural food sources:* Eggs (yolk) & oily fish, such as salmon, sardines & mackerel. Obviously be aware of your food intolerance or allergies as talked about earlier in this book.

Taking Additional Fibre

Fibre is the easiest way to ensure that your digestive system is flushing effectively & thoroughly.

Ideally, after reading this far you should be eating a lot more protein & taking a few specific supplements, so fiber is a healthy balance for movement of food through your digestive system.

An easy & extremely healthy way of taking in more fibre is to juice. Juicing vegetables as talked about earlier is extremely good for you.

It would be hard to ingest the optimal amount of vegetables per day by simply eating them! That's a lot of veg. So juicing provides a very simple way of drinking them. You get all the nutritional benefits without the chewing!

On top of which your digestive system doesn't have to work hard digesting (breaking down) the liquid so the vitamins & minerals are more easily absorbed.

I always recommend one to three juices per day to my clients. It's cheap & takes only a few minutes to prepare each juice.

If you cant cram a juice or two in to your day then I strongly suggest you supplement…

Fibrous Tips

- ***Good fibre supplements come in powder form.***

- ***How do you choose?*** Look for a trusted brand. Trial & error is the only way to tell if this supplement is a good match for your system. However, it's difficult to make a useless fibre supplement so you wont go far wrong with whichever brand you choose.

- ***How much do you take?*** You need about thirty grams per day: fifteen grams at breakfast & fifteen at dinner. You can take an additional fifteen grams at lunch without any adverse effects & possibly some additional positives. Fifteen grams is approximately one heaped tablespoon.

- ***How long do you take it for?*** You should never stop taking fibre, especially because you are now on a high-protein diet. The trick is to monitor your bowel movements, as we spoke about earlier. A bowel movement should occur three times a day, on average & should be an easy, pleasurable experience.

- ***Benefits include a clean colon,*** which dramatically improves your mental capacity due to the number of neuro-receptors located in your gut & a clean system. Fibre also reduces the risk for many diseases, especially colon cancer. It leads to a high-energy body & a faster metabolism & gives you more powerful fat-burning potential, the feeling of satiety (being full) & improved detoxification of xenoestrogens (foreign estrogens that can cause damage to your body)

- ***Natural food sources:*** Plants & green vegetables.

Fibre also helps stabilise your blood-sugar levels & supports keeping you at your goal weight once you reach it.

Choose from insoluble or soluble fibre. A good supplement company will provide both in appropriate amounts. Source a good company & they will guide you in the right direction.

The brand I recommend can be purchased through my website.

Chapter 16:
Plan to Achieve Now

When health is absent, wisdom cannot reveal itself, art cannot become manifest, strength cannot be exerted, wealth is useless, and reason is powerless.

—Herophiles

Launching yourself into a whole new way of life is only worth it if there are rewards—short- & long-term rewards.

The Principles of Optimalisn are guiding lights that direct you along the road of those rewards.

In this final chapter, I'll walk you through some last-minute knowledge & give you some resources to help you get started with your new health & fitness goals.

Benefit from Biosignature Technology...

What is BioSignature technology? It's a scientific method of achieving fat loss & gaining muscle that was developed by world-renowned strength & conditioning coach Charles Poliquin.

A caliper reading is taken from twelve points on your body. The combination of these points, plus your height & weight, determine your body fat percentage & lean muscle mass.

This is a form of hormonal profiling & a system that can target fat loss.

It is commonly believed that you cannot spot reduce fat—meaning that you cannot target fat loss to a specific area of your body.

BioSignature turns this theory on its head. Each assessment is kept on record so you can clearly see your results & progress. Your practitioner will clearly see where you have followed the guidelines to improve areas of your body.

The big benefits of BioSignature technology is that after your initial assessment, you receive a tailored plan on how to target & eliminate those stubborn areas that you have been struggling to reduce for years.

- A qualified technician tests twelve major sites with a pair of calipers (a metal pincher with a dial attached)

- These measurements are analysed so that you can better understand your body & the effect your lifestyle, exercise, diet & supplementation is having. Your hormones will create a *fat response to your body*. Where you lay down fat is related to your hormone balance. Through this system you have a way to highlight problem areas & the power to target them—specifically, correctly & effectively.

I highly recommend using BioSignature technology if you are serious about your health, fitness, physical appearance & sporting performance.

I offer BioSignature assessments through my website.

Alternatively go to www.poliquingroup.com & locate a BioSignature practitioner in your area.

The War on Fat

BioSignature testing is a highly useful weapon in the fight against fat. Essentially it informs you of what areas need the most focus.

This system grants you access to the quickest route to your goal. It's like having a map of your journey, when you have never been to your destination. It is that useful.

From your results, you'll receive guidance on the most effective steps to take to stimulate the quickest response from your body. A plan can be set up using this system, in combination with your blood tests, placing you in a strong position to win your war against fat.

Types of training & eating habits will also be addressed after your assessment. A skilled practitioner will deliver a considerable amount of information about you & your life within one fifteen-minute assessment.

Your body doesn't lie. The state of your body was reached through your lifestyle, exercise, nutrition & supplementation structure over the past weeks & years.

You will slowly but surely alter the shape of your body the more you apply the information you learn from this book.

Main Benefits

- The system identifies your blocking factors—the areas that need focus.
- It helps correct internal & external body imbalances.
- It helps you gain the results you want by establishing a qualified, personalised plan.
- You can refine it over time & perfect your body shape, your health & performance.

There has to be a sustainable way for you to track & improve your body. Otherwise it is easy to get sidetracked & complacent & forget about monitoring the things that really matter to your metabolism & in turn your body shape, not to mention your health.

In order to reach & maintain an optimal state of being, you need a support system. Every top athlete in the world has a coach. Every top singer, every musician on their way to the top had training from a professional.

My theory of Optimalism empowers you to become the physical, mental & emotional powerhouse you have always wanted to be. It enables you to be your best.

If you live in North West London, & would like a consultation, you can make contact through my website:
http://www.shapetrainer.co.uk/contact.php

Alternatively, you can find your local Bio-Signature Practitioner at:
http://www.poliquingroup.com/TrainerDirectory/FindaCoach
.aspx

Refine Yourself—Quickly!

Refinement is something that is enormously satisfying—& really the cherry on the cake for anyone living the Optimalism lifestyle.

Once you have lost the weight, built muscle & sorted out many of the health concerns that have sucked away your vitality in the past, your next step is to settle into your body, maintain it & continue to develop it further.

Everyday, you have the choice to improve yourself & the experience of your life. One solid way of doing this is to take your level of health to an all time high. That is what I have been coaching you toward throughout this book.

That is one of the gems of life... The opportunity to improve each & every day.

If you make conscious, repeated, quality effort, you will improve your body, mind, emotions & surroundings. It won't be instant & the rate of progress can sometimes seem frustrating but overall it will be worth it.

You must keep applying improved methods. Alter what you were doing, maybe only slightly. There is a perfect method for a period of time, which will take you to the next level. You may then need to alter that method to keep getting results.

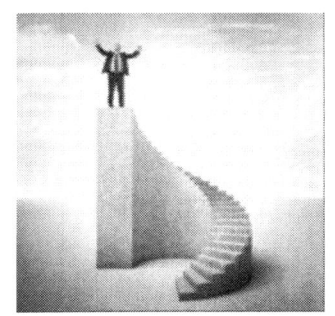

It is a virtual never-ending staircase toward greater health, vitality, happiness, fitness & success.

The type of person you are will be excited by the thought of this never-ending upward spiral.

You face issues head on. Find a solution. Improve that solution. Make it work. It is the underlying catalyst of all your success.

I respect that approach. Sometimes it is the only way to win.

I specifically wrote this book with the intention of directing you toward the right knowledge, in the right areas. This book contains some potent ideas & techniques.

I have attempted to squeeze concentrated information into the pages in the simplest & most easily digestible form so that you can benefit from it all.

To keep refining your progress, return to these pages, re-read the sections you know you are lacking in.

To help you further I have created a self-assessment report that you can complete for free.

I'll introduce you to this at the end of the book

Having Optimalsim Work For You

Imagine telling people that the way they live is all-wrong. Most people don't want to hear it. Then as they get older, symptoms of the faults in their lifestyle begin to appear.

They get worn out easily. They gain weight. They struggle to maintain relationships because work takes it out of them. In my opinion that is *no* way to live. Is there another way?

Optimalism & its Principles through LENS (lifestyle, exercise, nutrition, supplementation) works. I have used these principles for years & helped many of my clients recover from low level health, low fitness levels & low performance, using the systems outlined in this book.

But the only person who can really make it work is you. You decide what is right & what is wrong for your body, your mind & your lifestyle. Success may take a little sacrifice—you understand that better than most.

If you want a dynamic, healthy body alongside your career success, then you are going to have to work just as smart for it.

Notice I said *smart*, not *hard*. Anyone can slave away on a treadmill in a gym & hope the fat falls off. I'm here to show you there's an easier way.

As in business, you need a plan, a strategy. You also need a team of people behind you, feeding you the right insights & knowledge. Without that, the task at hand becomes infinitely harder.

Let the Principles of Optimalism stimulate your health & reshape your body from the inside out. After all of this time working for success, you can take a moment to consider the real wealth in life—your health.

Principle Exercise 24
Sharing Is Caring

I'd like to be a little cute at this point & use the word supplement in a different context. You see I have found that sharing is caring – even if you don't know who's listening!

By sharing your knowledge, just like I am sharing mine within this book, you help others.

By simply sharing your experience while walking your personal path to Optimalism you help others. Others then get the experience that someone cared enough to share invaluable information & insight with them.

You benefit them… & by benefitting them you benefit yourself.

You may be thinking 'So what's the point or how does that help me?'

Along my own personal journey of discovery I noticed a hidden jewel when it comes to continual progression. To help refine yourself over time, share what you learn, about yourself, about health, about vitality with others.

Share this book & what you learnt from it. When you share you inspire others, you get others working in the same way as you are. You encourage others to try on new techniques. Others say things in reply to your sharing that make you see a situation or technique in a different light.

***This will help to keep you on track, & bring others
in line with your progress***

*As I mentioned, long-term fitness is more easily achieved when you
are accountable & have a solid support system around you. That
means getting your friends, family, colleagues & strangers involved.*

*When you gain a new understanding share it. You may bring
clarity to someone else who then wants to work with you to create
another level of understanding. This process has no end.*

*So simply share what you learn. Try the techniques I've provided
within this book & share what works for you with others. It's that
simple.*

Principle 24
I Supplement Others

This principle is accessible at any point by giving your knowledge freely. Your knowledge base can be from any area of life. You have something to give – what you have learnt up to this point.

When you share what you know, you solidify the teaching in your own mind. You refine your understanding of it. You pass the knowledge on & gain a person(s) to work with.

By reading this book you now have an understanding of how to achieve your optimal state of being, how to increase your level of health & performance.

We've shed light over lifestyle applications, exercise selection, nutritional requirements & supplemental options.

You can share your journey as your understanding deepens. And let me tell you that the lifestyle of Optimalism is never ending. The depth of knowledge, understanding & potential progress is endless.

You can now begin to form your personal Health & Fitness Success Plan. Once you have formed this idea in your mind & begin to implement it, you will be able to begin sharing your expanding knowledge with others.

You'll refine your approach over time - Only then will you achieve your true personal best.

Only then will you achieve your optimal state of being & be able to share it with the world, in every way.

Conclusion

I've heard many times that, "You cannot have it all." Or "You cannot have your cake & eat it to". Why not?

I always say "What's the point in having a cake, if you can't eat it?" (As long as it's a gluten free, sugar free, low fat, protein cake, of course?!)

There are people who do have it all. I'm here to tell you that you can too. It's all about knowledge, balance & desire.

In my search for understanding of what it is to be optimal, what it is to reach an optimal state, what it means to live in an optimal state of being I discovered many truths, tips & hurdles to overcome.

This book is the result of that searching, trial & error. With it I hope to save you pain, frustration & most importantly – time.

When you begin to apply the principles of Optimalism, one by one, you'll start to notice a subtle shift. This upward shift will slowly but surely infiltrate your body, mind, emotions & performance.

Others will begin to notice something different about you. You'll be you, just even better. You'll notice that each day is less of a drag & more of a pull.

You see, when you are at optimal health you rise & shine rather than rise & whine. The day ahead appears as opportunity rather than routine.

I think what stops most from having this experience is knowledge. The knowledge that I have shared with you in this book. Each principle pulls you closer to your optimal state.

Most think that to be healthy requires hard work & too much planning. But the truth is that it really doesn't. It takes just as much effort to be unhealthy. The difference being that you simply feel worse when you're unhealthy.

When you are unhealthy you simply cannot enjoy life as much. That is a fact.

So the thought of hard work in the gym & a little preparation scares most people. We both know that if you want to achieve something extraordinary, whether it's in business or with your body, you need to *apply effort & focus in.*

Optimalism provides you the structure through which to focus. Apply the principles daily so that nothing can stop you.

That is how I have helped hundreds of highly successful people improve how they look, how they feel & how they perform for the better.

By focusing your efforts through these principles you will experience results like never before.

This is the end of the book, but the beginning of your heightened wellness journey. There is no greater reward from promoting life in your own body than experiencing life in ultra high definition.

With the right lifestyle, exercise, nutrition & supplementation principles, you can build a body to match your jaw-dropping career.

It's just good science.

Let's begin.

-Daniel Grant

Next Step: Don't risk putting this book down & doing nothing...

A Free Personal Health Report

I have created a free questionnaire for you – it will help you define which area of LENS you should focus on to bring about the greatest affect in the shortest possible time.

Once you've completed this simple survey about yourself you will instantly receive a report. This report will highlight your key focus areas & direct you where best to focus your energy for the quickest route to results.

It will provide you with some instant solutions to your highlighted areas that you can apply straight away.

The report provides you with direct access to your key steps toward achieving Optimalism in your life as quickly as possible.

This is a short cut to your optimal state. You can take the Optimalism Assessment & receive a free report, sent to your email shortly after, here:

www.LENSIndicator.com

About the Author

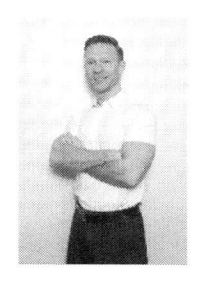

Daniel Grant

Author
Personal Health & Fitness Consultant
Creator of Optimalism

Daniel Grant is a body-shaping expert who has worked as a personal trainer for more than fifteen years.

He's helped numerous high-profile people reach and remain at their personal best amid their busy lifestyles. His seven-week program for stunning body transformations has proven itself time and time again.

A sports enthusiast and overall health and fitness addict, Daniel has expertise in numerous health and fitness disciplines. He is a BioSignature fat-loss system practitioner, CHEK practitioner, level-three holistic lifestyle coach, Reiki master, and body transformation specialist.

Daniel trained in Shiatsu as well as developing a deep understanding of how to cure low back pain as he consistently achieves success with low-back re-habilitation clients.

He has also co-developed iPhone fitness apps that put a personal trainer in your pocket.

Daniel's mission is to help you create your very own 'Greek God Body' and leave you feeling limitless.

Social Media Connections

Facebook Profile-
https://www.facebook.com/TheShapeTrainer.danielgrant

7Week-Body-Transformation Page-
https://www.facebook.com/7WeekBodyTransformation

LinkedIn:
ShapeTrainer Daniel Grant

Twitter:
@TheShapeTrainer

Instagram:
ShapeTrainer

References

Chapter 1

Dr Greenberg, Melanie, *The Best Quotes on Healthy Living*, http://www.psychologytoday.com/blog/the-mindful-self-express/201305/the-best-quotes-healthy-living

Leading a Healthy Life: Six Steps To Living Long and Staying Healthy, http://depts.washington.edu/uwcoe/healthtopics/healthylife.html

10 Tips For a Healthy Lifestyle, http://www.independent.co.uk/life-style/health-and-families/healthy-living/10-tips-for-a-healthy-lifestyle-783833.html

The Effects of a Non-Sedentary Workspace on Information Elaboration and Group Performance
Andrew P. Knight **&** Markus Baer
Published online before print June 12, 2014, doi:10.1177/1948550614538463Social Psychological and Personality Science June 12, 20141948550614538463

Ultradian Rhythms in Prolonged Human Performance
Peretz Lavie, Jacob Zomer, and Daniel Gopher
Institute of Technology
Haifa, Israel

Dopamine
http://www.bps.org.uk/news/study-questions-dopamines-part-adhd

Dr. Lachman, the Manhattan Project of middle age, an <u>enormous study</u> titled Midlife in the United States, or Midus.

Pelvic Floor and Prostrate Cancer
http://www.theherald.com.au/story/2525555/mens-pelvic-floor-exercises-could-prevent-prostate-related-incontinence/

Chapter 2

Stress Quotes, BrainyQuote, http://www.brainyquote.com/quotes/keywords/stress.html

Weekly Exercise Requirements:
http://www.acsm.org/about-acsm/media-room/news-releases/2011/08/01/acsm-issues-new-recommendations-on-quantity-and-quality-of-exercise

The Shocking Truth About Drinking Tap Water, http://martinwhitaker.co.uk/the-truth-about-drinking-tap-water/

Chan, Amanda, *Stress Health Effects: 10 Scary Things It's*

Doing To Your Body, http://www.huffingtonpost.com/2013/02/04/stress-health-effects-cancer-immune-system_n_2599551.html

Haak, Emma, *The Science of Stress: 5 Things Worrying Is Doing To Your Body,* http://www.oprah.com/spirit/Science-of-Stress-What-Stress-Does-to-Your-Body

The Effects of a Non-Sedentary Workspace on Information Elaboration and Group Performance
Andrew P. Knight
Markus Baer
Washington University in St. Louis, MO, USA

Published online before print June 12, 2014, doi:10.1177/194855 0614538463 Social Psychological and Personality Science **June 12, 2014**1948550614538463

Brain Body Stress
https://books.google.co.uk/books?hl=en&lr=&id=AwvS1kzQuY8C&oi
=fnd&pg=PP1&dq=body+language+and+stress&ots=a7it-WCPfB&sig
=h5ZSKvHIZv97_CBWpW94riz25AM#v=onepage&q&f=false

Surrounded by pollution
http://www.nrdc.org/health/

Pg. 43
[1] Are vacations good for your health? The 9-year mortality experience
after the multiple risk factor intervention trial.
http://www.ncbi.nlm.nih.gov/pubmed/11020089

Chapter 3

Stress Relief Quotes: 16 Calming Phrases To Reduce Anxiety,
http://www.huffingtonpost.com/2012/08/28/stress-relief-quotes-
oasis-2012_n_1836145.html

How To Rid Yourself of Anxiety For Good,
http://www.livestressfreelifestyle.com/anxiety/
how-to-rid-yourself-of-anxiety-for-good/

Csatari, Jeff, *Where Stress Hides*, http://www.menshealth.com/health/
stress-relief-tips

Pg. 50
[2] "Mindfullness-based Stress Reduction Helps Lower
Blood Pressure Study Finds," http://www.sciencedaily.com/
releases/2013/10/131015094436.htm

Pg. 50
[1] Carolyn Aldwin, Nuoo-Ting Molitor, "Do Stress Trajectories Predict Mortality in Older Men? Longitudinal Findings from the VA Normative Aging Study," *Journal of Aging Research*, http://www.hindawi.com/journals/jar/2011/896109/.

Pg70
Even in cool laboratory conditions, maximal aerobic power (VO2max) decreases by about 5% when persons experience fluid losses equivalent to 3% of body mass or more (Pinchan et al. 1988). http://www.humankinetics.com/products/all-products/Sport-Nutrition---2nd-Edition

[1] "Mindfullness-based Stress Reduction Helps Lower Blood Pressure Study Finds," http://www.sciencedaily.com/releases/2013/10/131015094436.htm

http://www.sleepeducation.com/news/2012/07/05/sleep-loss-triggers-stress-like-immune-response. American Academy of Sleep Medicine | Jul 04, 2012

Chapter 4

Deborah Day Quotes, Goodreads, http://www.goodreads.com/author/quotes/1438286.Deborah_Day

Murphy, Frederique, *7 Strategies To Control Your Thoughts (And Not The Other Way Around),* http://mountainmovingmindset.com/blog/?p=1173

Replantaion at eMedicine. http://en.wikipedia.org/wiki/EMedicine

Chapter 5

Fitness Quotes, BrainyQuote,
http://www.brainyquote.com/quotes/topics/topic_fitness.html

Pg112 Weight training improves insulin sensitivity
http://care.diabetesjournals.org/content/21/8/1353.abstract

pg112 Weight training increases longevity.
http://www.cdc.gov/physicalactivity/growingstronger/why/

pg 112
What Is Oxidative Stress?, http://www.news-medical.net/health/
What-is-Oxidative-Stress.aspx

Dr Weil, Andrew, *Stumped By Oxidative Stress,*
http://www.drweil.com/drw/u/QAA400537/Stumped-by-
Oxidative-Stress.html

Gluhareff, David, *Why Weight Training,*
http://www.bodybuilding.com/fun/gluhareff4.htm

Mueller, Jen, *Why Strength Training Is a Must For Everyone,*
http://www.sparkpeople.com/resource/fitness_articles.asp?id=364

Robertson, Mike, *The Truth About Weight Training vs. Cardio,*
http://www.huffingtonpost.com/livestrongcom/the-truth-about-
weight-training-vs-cardio_b_894936.html

Dr Mercola, *Extreme Endurance Cardio May Do More Harm Than
Good,* http://fitness.mercola.com/sites/fitness/archive/2012/12/21/
extreme-endurance-cardio.aspx

Chapter 6

Lee Haney, BrainyQuotes,
http://www.brainyquote.com/quotes/quotes/l/leehaney295632.html
Your Online Guide To Weight Training Exercise, http://www.weight-training-exercises.com/

Exercise Guides, http://www.bodybuilding.com/exercises/

Strength Training Exercises, http://www.mydr.com.au/sports-fitness/strength-training-exercises

Pelvic floor exercises for women
http://www.ncbi.nlm.nih.gov/pubmed/25648223

Chapter 7

Exercise Quotes, BrainyQuote,
http://www.brainyquote.com/quotes/keywords/exercise.html

Schirm, Matthew, *What Muscles Do Squats Target?,*
http://www.livestrong.com/
article/416344-what-muscles-do-squats-work-out/

Deadlift, Wikipedia, http://en.wikipedia.org/wiki/Deadlift

Kamb, Steve, *Deadlift – The Ultimate Exercise. Not Just For*

Zombies, http://www.nerdfitness.com/blog/2009/07/22/
deadlift-the-ultimate-exercise-not-just-for-zombies/

Johnson, Jolie, *What Muscles Does a Deadlift
Work Out,* http://www.livestrong.com/
article/416598-what-muscles-does-a-deadlift-work-out/

Mark, *Deadlifts and Ten Unique Benefits You Should Know About,*
http://trainheavy.com/people/ten-unique-benefits-of-the-deadlift/
Dr Mercola, *Squats: 8 Reasons To Do This Misunderstood Exercise,*
http://fitness.mercola.com/sites/fitness/archive/2012/05/25/darin-
steen-demonstrates-the-perfect-squat.aspx

Perry, Marc, *How To Squat: 7 Tips For Proper Form
and Technique,* http://www.builtlean.com/2010/07/20/
how-to-do-proper-squat-technique/

Kamb, Steve, *Why You Need Squats In Your Workout And How To
Do Them Right,* http://www.nerdfitness.com/blog/2009/07/08/
why-you-need-squats-in-your-workout-and-how-to-do-them-right/

Squat (exercise), Wikipedia, http://en.wikipedia.org/wiki/
Squat_(exercise)

Mehdi, *How To Barbell Row: 7 Tips To Master Proper Barbell Row
Form,* http://stronglifts.com/how-to-master-barbell-row-technique/

Bent-Over Row, Wikipedia, http://en.wikipedia.org/wiki/Bent-over_row

Bench Press, Wikipedia, http://en.wikipedia.org/wiki/Bench_press

Smith, Jim, *Bench Press 101,* http://www.schwarzenegger.com/fitness/
post/bench-press-101

Smith, Jim, *8 Great Tips For a Better Bench Press,*
http://www.muscleandfitness.com/workouts/
chest-exercises/8-great-tips-better-bench-press

Henriques, Tim, *Why The Bench Press Is The Best Exercise,*
http://www.t-nation.com/free_online_article/most_recent/
why_the_bench_press_is_the_best_exercise

The Fitness Benefits of Pullups, http://www.fitday.com/fitness-articles/fitness/exercises/the-fitness-benefits-of-pullups.html#b

Rail, Kevin, *Benefits of Pull-Ups*, http://www.livestrong.com/article/90190-benefits-pullups/

Exercise Guides – Abdominal Exercises, http://www.bodybuilding.com/exercises/finder/lookup/filter/muscle/id/13/muscle/abdominals

How Core Fitness Exercise Benefits The Entire Body, http://www.fitday.com/fitness-articles/fitness/body-building/how-core-fitness-exercise-benefits-the-entire-body.html#b

Bayer, Jeff, *The Truth About Abdominal Training*, http://uk.askmen.com/sports/bodybuilding_200/202_fitness_tip.html

Pull-Ups (exercise), Wikipedia, http://en.wikipedia.org/wiki/Pull-up_(exercise)
Melton, Philip, *The Importance of Pull-Ups*, http://www.livinghealthy360.com/index.php/the-importance-of-pull-ups-75598/

The Fitness Benefits of Pullups, http://www.fitday.com/fitness-articles/fitness/exercises/the-fitness-benefits-of-pullups.html#b

Henriques, Time, *Why The Bench Press Is The Best Exercise*, http://www.t-nation.com/free_online_article/most_recent/why_the_bench_press_is_the_best_exercise

Why Bench Press Is Important, http://www.fitnessquests.com/2010/04/why-bench-press-is-important.html

Quinene, Paula, *What Are The Benefits of Bench Press*, http://www.livestrong.com/article/98767-benefits-bench-presses/

Dip (exercise), Wikipedia, http://en.wikipedia.org/wiki/
Dip_(exercise)

151 Importance of lean muscle mass
http://www.ncbi.nlm.nih.gov/pubmed/22030953

151 Lean mass reduces cvd in older women
http://www.ncbi.nlm.nih.gov/pubmed/24997614

151 Lean mass improves blood pressure
http://www.ncbi.nlm.nih.gov/pubmed/24707476

Chapter 8

Exercise Quotes, BrainyQuote,
http://www.brainyquote.com/quotes/keywords/exercise.html
Eberhardt, Tanya, *Definition of Reps and Sets*, http://www.livestrong.
com/article/153380-definition-of-reps-sets/

De Salles, BF, Simao, R, Miranda, F, *Rest Interval Between Sets in
Strength Training*, http://www.ncbi.nlm.nih.gov/pubmed/19691365

Hughes, Ryan, *Ask The Pro Trainer*, http://www.bodybuilding.com/fun/
ask-the-pro-trainer-how-important-is-the-number-of-reps-i-do.html

*Strong Science – Research On The Ideal Rep Range and Sets To
Maximize Results*, http://www.simplyshredded.com/strong-science-
research-on-the-ideal-rep-range-number-of-sets-to-maximize-
results.html

Double Crunch, http://randomabs.com/exercises/
howto/?show=Double_Crunch

Pushups, http://www.bodybuilding.com/exercises/detail/view/name/
pushups

Instructions, http://www.exrx.net/WeightExercises/Brachioradialis/BBReverseCurl.html

Bodyweight Squat, http://www.acefitness.org/acefit/fitness_programs_exercise_library_details.aspx?exerciseid=135

Dip (exercise), Wikipedia, http://en.wikipedia.org/wiki/Dip_(exercise) *Dips – Triceps Version,* http://www.bodybuilding.com/exercises/detail/view/name/dips-triceps-version

Training Times For Optimal Health Response
http://www.ncbi.nlm.nih.gov/pubmed/24715614
http://www.ncbi.nlm.nih.gov/pubmed/25144130

Muscle atrophy
http://ajcn.nutrition.org/content/91/4/1123S.full
http://www.livestrong.com/article/383660-how-fast-do-you-lose-muscle-by-not-training/

Chapter 9

Quotes About Nutrition, http://www.goodreads.com/quotes/tag/nutrition

Latest Obesity Stats For England Are Alarming,
http://www.nhs.uk/news/2013/02February/Pages/Latest-obesity-stats-for-England-are-alarming-reading.aspx

Statistics on Obesity, Physical Activity and Diet England, 2013,
http://www.bhfactive.org.uk/userfiles/Documents/obes-phys-acti-diet-eng-2013-rep.pdf

Your gut the second brain
http://www.scientificamerican.com/article/gut-second-brain/

Malnutrition: UK's Silent Killer,
http://www.thenacc.co.uk/assets/downloads/144/
Malnutrition%20-%20UKs%20silent%20killer.pdf

Malnutrition, http://www.nhs.uk/conditions/Malnutrition/Pages/
Introduction.aspx

Malnutrition – Overcoming The Problem,
http://www.bda.uk.com/foodfacts/MalnutritionFactSheet.pdf

NHS calorie intake
http://www.nhs.uk/chq/pages/1126.aspx?categoryid=51

Dr Weil, Andrew, *Anti-Inflammatory Diet and Pyramid,*
http://www.drweil.com/drw/u/ART02012/anti-inflammatory-diet
Pevzner, Holly, *10 Ways To Reduce Inflammation,*
http://www.eatingwell.com/nutrition_health/
nutrition_news_information/10_ways_to_reduce_inflammation

Orthodontics & Facial Spacing Alterations relating to diet
[3] http://www.pnas.org/search?fulltext=Noreen+von+Cram
on-Taubadel&submit=yes&x=0&y=0
[2] http://www.strategyr.com/Orthodontic_Supplies_Market_
Report.asp
[3] http://www.statista.com/topics/863/fast-food/

Chapter 10

Quotes About Nutrition, Goodreads, http://www.goodreads.com/
quotes/tag/nutrition

Mehdi, *Protein 101: How Much Do You Need and
Best Sources of Protein,* http://stronglifts.com/
protein-daily-needs-myths-best-sources-protein/

O'Donnell, Mike, *The Truth on How Much Protein You Really Need Per Day To Build Muscle,* http://www.theiflife.com/ how-much-protein-per-day-build-muscle/

Walker, Jennifer, *Protein Up Your Detox*, http://www.alive.com/ articles/view/20051/protein_up_your_detox

Wilson, Pamela, *The Low-GI Diet Explained*, http://health.ninemsn. com.au/dietandnutrition/nutrition/693899/the-low-gi-diet

Low Glycemic Foods, Explained, http://www.huffingtonpost. com/2012/06/27/low-glycemic-foods-diet_n_1630893.html

Raffetto, Meri, *Benefits of a Low-Glycemic Diet,* http://www.dummies. com/how-to/content/benefits-of-a-lowglycemic-diet.html

4 Reasons To Eat Low GI Foods, http://www.besthealthmag.ca/ eat-well/healthy-eating/4-reasons-to-eat-low-gi-foods

Food Storage Containers, http://www.nrdc.org/living/shoppingwise/ food-storage-containers.asp

Water Consumption and productivity levels
http://www.ncbi.nlm.nih.gov/pubmed/20974676
http://www.naturalhydrationcouncil.org.uk/wp-content/ uploads/2012/06/Hydration-at-Work.pdf

Dr Hoffman, Matthew, Pots, Pans, and Plastics: A Shoppers Guide To Food Safety, http://www.webmd.com/food-recipes/features/ cookware-plastics-shoppers-guide-to-food-safety

Boggan, Steve, *Poisoned By Plastic: Chemicals in Water Bottles and Food Packaging Have Been Linked To Infertility and Birth*

Defects. Scaremongering, or The Truth?,
http://www.dailymail.co.uk/health/article-2157423/

Poisoned-plastic-Chemicals-water-bottles-food-packaging-linked-infertility-birth-defects-Scaremongering-truth.html

Sawyer, Jodi, Why Is Fibre So Important, http://www.doctoroz.com/blog/jodi-sawyer-rn/why-fiber-so-important

Why Is Fibre Important, http://www.nhs.uk/chq/pages/1141.aspx?categoryid=51

Atkinson, Louise, *Healthy Signs: How To Monitor Your Bowel Movements,* http://www.dailymail.co.uk/health/article-1307575/Healthy-signs-How-monitor-bowel-movements.html

Bowel Function, http://www.myfitnesspal.com/topics/show/20956-bowel-function

Fibre and cholesterol
http://www.ncbi.nlm.nih.gov/pubmed/25346913

The New Food Pyramid, http://www.washingtonpost.com/wp-srv/nation/daily/graphics/diet_042005.html

Glycemic Index and Load
http://www.ncbi.nlm.nih.gov/pubmed/17344493
http://www.hsph.harvard.edu/nutritionsource/carbohydrates/carbohydrates-and-blood-sugar/

Over production of Insulin damages cells
http://www.sciencedaily.com/releases/2007/07/070719141139.htm

Food Pyramid – Reduce Inflammation, http://simplyfantasticbooks.com/2013/05/30/food-pyramid-reduce-inflammation/

Breakfast Cereal Study
file:///Users/danielgrant/Downloads/NOC_Extruder.pdf

Diabetes Rates
http://www.diabetes.org.uk/About_us/What-we-say/Statistics/
Diabetes-in-the-UK-2013-Key-statistics-on-diabetes/

Chapter 11

Edward Group, *The 50 Best Quotes About Health and Nutrition*,
http://www.lewrockwell.com/2011/07/edward-group/
the-50-best-quotes-about-health-nutrition/

Doherty, Elissa, *Low Carb/High Protein Diets*, http://www.bodyandsoul
.com.au/weight+loss/diets/low+carb+high+protein+diets,8263

The Protein Power Diet, http://www.webmd.com/diet/
protein-power-what-it-is

Rieske, Kent, *Scientific Proof Carbohydrates Cause Disease*,
http://articles.mercola.com/sites/articles/archive/2004/01/03/
carbohydrates-age.aspx

Dr Oz, *Do Carbs Cause Alzheimer's*, http://www.doctoroz.com/
episode/do-carbs-cause-alzheimers
General Nutrition, http://www.nutrition.org.uk/

How Much Should I Eat?, http://www.medicalnewstoday.com/
articles/219305.php

Healthy Eating, http://www.nhs.uk/livewell/healthy-eating/Pages/
Healthyeating.aspx

Cut Down On Your Calories, http://www.nhs.uk/Livewell/Goodfood/
Pages/eat-less.aspx#you

What Are Calories? What Is a Calorie, http://www.medicalnewstoday.
com/articles/263028.php

Mack, Stan, *Why Does The Human Body Need Food To Survive?*, http://www.livestrong.com/article/466201-why-does-the-human-body-need-food-to-survive/

Katz, David, *Mom Was Right: You Are What You Eat*, http://www.nbcnews.com/id/35350889/#.UrWNvfQW0Ww

Chapter 12

Food Quotes, http://www.brainyquote.com/quotes/topics/topic_food.html

Choosing Healthy Fats, http://www.helpguide.org/life/healthy_diet_fats.htm

14 Best Vegan and Vegetarian Protein Sources, http://www.health.com/health/gallery/0,,20718479_7,00.html

What Foods To Eat on a Low-Carb Diet, http://lowcarbdiets.about.com/od/whattoeat/

Dolson, Laura, *Low-Carb Fruit List: The Best and The Worst*

Fruits, http://lowcarbdiets.about.com/od/whattoeat/a/whatfruit.htm

Food as Fuel: Before, During and After Workouts, http://www.heart.org/HEARTORG/GettingHealthy/PhysicalActivity/Food-as-Fuel-Before-During-and-After-

Workouts_UCM_436451_Article.jsp#
How To Create a Bodybuilding Diet, http://www.muscleandstrength.com/articles/how-to-create-a-bodybuilding-diet.html

Roussell, Mike, *Meal Plan For Every Guy*, http://www.bodybuilding.com/fun/meal-plan-for-every-guy.html

Top 10 Foods Highest in Protein, http://www.healthaliciousness.com/articles/foods-highest-in-protein.php

Top 10 Best and Worst Protein Sources (Vegetarians Take Note), http://www.marksdailyapple.com/top-ten-protein-sources/#axzz2o7I38OZ2

Chapter 13

Quotes About Supplements, Goodreadshttp://www.goodreads.com/quotes/tag/supplements Spano, Marie, *Bodybuilding Helps You Choose The Right Supplement*, http://www.bodybuilding.com/fun/how-bodybuilding-helps-you-choose-the-right-supplements.html

Questions To Ask Before Taking Vitamin and Mineral Supplements, http://www.nutrition.gov/dietary-supplements/questions-ask-taking-vitamin-and-mineral-supplements

Decrease in Nutritional Values
http://hortsci.ashspublications.org/content/44/1/15.full
http://www.scientificamerican.com/article/soil-depletion-and-nutrition-loss/

Age of our food
http://www.foodrenegade.com/your-apples-year-old/

BPA In Water Bottles
http://www.dailymail.co.uk/health/article-2157423/Poisoned-plastic-Chemicals-water-bottles-food-packaging-linked-infertility-birth-defects-Scaremongering-truth.html

Dry Cleaning Chemicals
http://www.webmd.com/cancer/news/20100209/dry-cleaning-chemical-likely-causes-cancer
http://www.naturalnews.com/023365_health_cleaning_dry.html

Dietary Supplements: What You Need To Know, http://ods.od.nih.gov/
HealthInformation/DS_WhatYouNeedToKnow.aspx

Population Nutrient Deficiencies
http://www.cdc.gov/media/releases/2012/p0402_vitamins_nutrients.html

*Vitamin Pills Are a Waste of Money, Offer No Health Benefits and
Could Be harmful, Study,* http://www.independent.co.uk/life-style/
health-and-families/health-news/vitamin-pills-are-a-waste-of-money-
offer-no-health-benefits-and-could-be-harmful--study-9010303.html

Dr Oz's *Ultimate Supplement Checklist,* http://www.doctoroz.com/
videos/dr-ozs-ultimate-supplement-checklist

Chapter 14

Good Health Quotes, BrainyQuote,
http://www.brainyquote.com/quotes/keywords/good_health.html

Horton, Tony, *Supplement Your Diet,* http://uk.askmen.com/sports/
foodcourt/supplement-your-diet.html

Henderson, Lynne, Irving, Karen, Gregory, Jan, *The National Diet
and Nutrition Survey: Adults Aged 19 To 64 Years,* http://www.food.
gov.uk/multimedia/pdfs/ndnsv3.pdf

Starling, Shane, *Supplements - Who Needs Them? Er Around 85%
of Working Adults, Says Stats,* http://www.nutraingredients.com/
Industry/Supplements-Who-needs-them-Er-around-85-of-working-
adults-say-stats

Why Do We Need Supplements?, http://stayhealthyandwell.com/
why-do-we-need-supplements/

Dr Hyman, Mark, *Do You Need Nutritional Supplements,*
http://drhyman.com/blog/2010/12/17/
do-you-need-nutritional-supplements/

Use nutritional supplements to boost immune system
http://www.ncbi.nlm.nih.gov/pubmed/24281460

Why Getting Your Nutrition Only From Food Is a Bad Idea,
http://www.bulletproofexec.com/why-you-need-supplements/
Poliquin, Charles, 10 Very Good Reasons For you To Take Supplements,
http://www.poliquingroup.com/Tips/tabid/130/entryid/357/10-very-good-reasons-for-you-to-take-supplements.aspx

Chapter 15

Sachem, John, *35 Fitness and Health Quotes,* http://voices.yahoo.com/35-fitness-health-quotes-5984338.html?cat=5

Live Five Years Longer With A Multivitamin
http://www.ncbi.nlm.nih.gov/pubmed/19279081

Rider, Sam, *Amino Acids? Should You Take Them?,*
http://www.mensfitness.co.uk/nutrition/supplements/1155/amino-acids-should-you-take-them
4 Possible Amino Acid Side Effects, http://www.fitday.com/fitness-articles/nutrition/vitamins-minerals/4-possible-amino-acid-side-effects.html#b

American Heart Association Recommendations of omega-3
http://www.heart.org/HEARTORG/GettingHealthy/NutritionCenter/HealthyDietGoals/Fish-and-Omega-3-Fatty-Acids_UCM_303248_Article.jsp

Krans, Brian, *Why Men Should Avoid Fish Oil*
Supplements, http://www.healthline.com/health-news/again-why-men-should-avoid-fish-oil-071113

Leyva, John, *Fish Oil Supplements 101: Fat Loss Benefits, Function and Dosage,* http://www.builtlean.com/2012/01/19/fish-oil-supplements/

Inflammation, Omega6 to Omega3 consumption
http://umm.edu/health/medical/altmed/supplement/
omega3-fatty-acids

American Heart Association Recommendation
http://www.heart.org/HEARTORG/GettingHealthy/NutritionCenter/
HealthyDietGoals/Fish-and-Omega-3-Fatty-Acids_UCM_303248_
Article.jsp

Fish Oil Sales
http://newhope360.com/breaking-news/
global-fish-oil-market-reach-33-billion-2020-researchers-say

Fish Oil and Body Composition
http://www.ncbi.nlm.nih.gov/pubmed/17490962

Fish Oil Alzheimer's
http://www.ncbi.nlm.nih.gov/pubmed/24954371

Fish Oil Bipolar & Brain
http://edition.cnn.com/2011/HEALTH/03/07/US.highest.bipolar.rates/

Vitamin D Replacement Improves Muscle Efficiency,
http://www.sciencedaily.com/releases/2013/03/130317221446.htm

Vitamin D and skeletal muscle
http://www.ncbi.nlm.nih.gov/pubmed/24488588
http://www.ncbi.nlm.nih.gov/pubmed/24179588

Vitamin D and mood
http://www.ncbi.nlm.nih.gov/pubmed/24488588
http://www.ncbi.nlm.nih.gov/pubmed/24179588

Vitamin D and SAD
http://www.ncbi.nlm.nih.gov/pubmed/23475735

Vitamin D and mineral absorption
http://www.ncbi.nlm.nih.gov/pubmed/25270233

D3 SAD
http://www.ncbi.nlm.nih.gov/pubmed/9539254

D3 Osteoporosis
http://link.springer.com/article/10.1007/BF00305521

Bone Density & Fractures
http://www.nejm.org/doi/full/10.1056/NEJM199709043371003

Autoimmune disease
http://www.aarda.org/autoimmune-information/autoimmune-statistics/

Immune Boosting D3
http://www.ncbi.nlm.nih.gov/pmc/articles/PMC3051848/

Harvard Article & Studies
http://www.hsph.harvard.edu/nutritionsource/vitamin-d/

D3 and Cancers, prevention
http://www.ncbi.nlm.nih.gov/pubmed/23239153
http://www.ncbi.nlm.nih.gov/pubmed/22508710
http://www.ncbi.nlm.nih.gov/pubmed/21724580
http://www.ncbi.nlm.nih.gov/pubmed/22939886
http://www.ncbi.nlm.nih.gov/pubmed/22801352

Health Claims About Vitamin D Explained, http://www.nhs.uk/
news/2013/06June/Pages/health-claims-about-vitamin-D-examined.aspx

Glutamine, WebMD, http://www.webmd.com/vitamins-supplements/
ingredientmono-878-

GLUTAMINE.aspx?activeIngredientId=878&activeIngredientName=
GLUTAMINE

Is Glutamine an Effective Supplement?, http://www.bodybuilding.
com/fun/glutamine_effectiveness.htm

Fibre and Fibre Supplements, http://www.patient.co.uk/health/
fibre-and-fibre-supplements

Chapter 16

Top 21 Health and Fitness Quotes, http://www.movemequotes.com/
top-21-health-and-fitness-quotes/

Poliquin BioSignature Modulation Level 1, http://www.poliquingroup.
com/Education/Biosignature/BiosignatureLevelOne.aspx

BioSignature Program, http://www.mybiosignature.com.au/
biosignature-program.html

Agu, Joseph, *An Objective Look at Biosignature
Modulation Part 1*, http://josephagu.com/2012/05/03/
an-objective-look-at-biosignature-modulation-part-1/

Made in the USA
Charleston, SC
03 April 2016